EARLY PRAISE!

"For those ready to move up to integrating behavioral health in primary care, this book should be the first stop. It is easy to read, comprehensive, and extremely practical—down to the level of job descriptions, worksheets, staffing ratios, and templates. The business and finance sections are easy to understand yet sophisticated—they should be required reading for all leaders working in primary care. These authors have produced something of real value. Bravo, and Thank You!"

Frank Verloin deGruy III, MD, MSFM
Woodward-Chisholm Professor and Chair
Department of Family Medicine
University of Colorado School of Medicine
Aurora, CO

"A welcome and timely resource for organizations looking to engage in integrated behavioral healthcare. It summarizes the published literature, information from case studies, and the authors' experiences from years in the field. Written in a concise, user-friendly format which will guide you step-by-step through the implementation process. I wish that this book existed years ago when KP started the integration journey."

Andrew Bertagnolli, PhD
Senior Manager—Integrated Behavioral Health Care Management Institute
Kaiser Permanente
Oakland, CA

"Physicians know that clinical outcomes can be improved by managing behavioral health comorbidities along with physical illnesses. But where do physicians and medical practices start?

Kent Corso and his distinguished co-authors give us the roadmap in *Integrating Behavioral Health Into the Medical Home: A Rapid Implementation Guide*. The book is well organized and provides a brilliant set of new tools to assess which service delivery model is right for your organization, how to master personnel selection and training of staff members, and a step-by-step guide on how to achieve the return on investment required to get the buy-in from your practice stakeholders."

Kevin Pho, MD
Founder, www.kevinmd.com
Nashua, NH

"Available at just the right time, this 'bottom line up front' book provides concise guidance for healthcare companies seeking to integrate behavioral health services into primary care. The authors provide a variety of forms to assist with selection of a service delivery model, develop a business plan, and evaluate return on investment. It concludes with a variety of case studies and exemplars to assure reader understanding and confidence in moving forward. Bravo!"

Patricia J. Robinson, PhD
Director of Training and Program Evaluation
Mountainview Consulting Group
Portland, OR

"I am tremendously excited to share this short book with all of my colleagues who are striving to establish and improve their own Primary Care Medical Home via integrating behavioral health—which means about everyone I know! The experienced authors achieve this book's stated purpose as 'A Rapid Implementation Guide' with succinct practical summaries of key points highlighted at the start of each chapter and often followed by easily understood appendices. This book is well referenced and written to help all of us, from novices to experienced pioneers."

Macaran (Mac) Baird, MD, MS
Professor and Chair, Department of Family Medicine and Community Health
University of Minnesota Medical School
Minneapolis, MN

"Just in the nick of time with healthcare reform, Corso, Hunter, Dahl, Kallenberg, and Manson bring us an eminently readable, highly practical manual to guide the process of integrating behavioral into physical healthcare. Healthcare reform provides the guidelines, this book provides invaluable blueprints that can be adapted to your context. It's even occasionally funny!

We live in a period of rapid change in healthcare; new financing incents comprehensive integrated care without providing guidance about how to make the care a practical reality. This essential book fills that gap—everything from integrated care models, financing, personnel, skill development, and exemplars."

Susan H McDaniel, PhD ABPP
Dr. Laurie Sands Distinguished Professor of Families & Health
Director, Institute for the Family, Department of Psychiatry
Associate Chair of Family Medicine
University of Rochester Medical Center
Rochester, NY

"We all have a neck connecting our head and body. This means every aspect of physical health is influenced by our minds. Addressing either physical health or mental health without integrating the two leads to failure—something we can't afford to have happen. *Integrating Behavioral Health into the Medical Home: A Rapid Implementation Guide* is the tool everyone needs in order to facilitate truly integrated healthcare—a must read!!"

Paul Grundy, MD, MPH
IBM's Global Director of Healthcare Transformation
President, Patient-Centered Primary Care Collaborative
Hopewell Junction, NY

"As momentum gains to truly embrace patient-centered healthcare, this how-to book is an essential component of your performance improvement library. Use *Integrating Behavioral Health into the Medical Home: A Rapid Implementation Guide* to architect your medical practice into a medical home successfully serving the whole person."

Elizabeth W. Woodcock, MBA, FACMPE, CPC
Author, *PCMH Policies and Procedures Guidebook*
Woodcock & Associates
Atlanta, GA

"*Integrating Behavioral Health into Medical Homes* is a comprehensive guide to providing holistic care to patients. The authors have covered every essential question on team-based healthcare delivery: what to do, why and how to do it. The 'Bottom Line, Up Front' feature at the beginning of each chapter makes this well-referenced and evidence-based book exceptionally easy to navigate. An invaluable guide to the concepts and practice of integrated behavioral healthcare."

Joseph P. Napora, PhD
Johns Hopkins Comprehensive Diabetes Center
Author, *Stress-Free Diabetes: Your Guide to Health and Happiness*
Baltimore, MD

"Most patients who are depressed or anxious or who need mental health treatment start at their primary care office. Most never get to a psychiatrist—they are treated by their PCP. Adding an organized behavioral health component will improve patient care and provide support for the primary care clinician. This book provides an invaluable, specific road map for practices."

Betsy Nicoletti, MS, CPC
Founder, www.Codapedia.com
Author, *The Field Guide to Physician Coding, 3rd Edition*
Northampton, MA

INTEGRATING BEHAVIORAL HEALTH INTO THE MEDICAL HOME:
A Rapid Implementation Guide

Kent A. Corso, PsyD, BCBA-D
Christopher L. Hunter, PhD, ABPP
Owen Dahl, MBA, FACHE, LSSMBB,
Gene A. Kallenberg, MD
Lesley Manson, PsyD

GREENBRANCH PUBLISHING
Phoenix, Maryland

Copyright © 2016 by Greenbranch Publishing, LLC
ISBN: 978-0-9962584-6-3
eISBN: 978-0-9962584-7-0

PO Box 208
Phoenix, MD 21131
Phone: (800) 933-3711
Fax: (410) 329-1510
Email: info@greenbranch.com
Websites: www.greenbranch.com, www.mpmnetwork.com, www.soundpractice.net, www.codapedia.com

All rights reserved. No part of this book shall be reproduced, stored in a retrieval system, or transmitted by any means, i.e. electronic, mechanical, photocopying, recording, or otherwise, without written permission of the publisher. Please do not participate in or encourage piracy of copyrighted materials in violation of the authors' rights. Purchase only authorized editions. Routine photocopying or electronic distribution to others is a copyright violation. Please notify us immediately at (800) 933-3711 if you have received any unauthorized editorial from this book.

No patent liability is assumed with respect to the use of the information contained herein. Although every precaution has been taken in the preparation of this book, the publisher and the authors assume no responsibility for errors or omissions. Nor is any liability assumed from damages resulting from the use of the information contained herein. For information, Greenbranch Publishing, PO Box 208, Phoenix, MD 21131.

This book includes representations of the author's personal experiences and do not reflect actual patients or medical situations.

This book is not intended as a substitute for the medical advice of physicians. The reader should regularly consult a physician in matters relating to his/her health and particularly with respect to any symptoms that may require diagnosis or medical attention.

The strategies contained herein may not be suitable for every situation. This publication is designed to provide general medical practice management information and is sold with the understanding that neither the author nor the publisher is engaged in rendering legal, accounting, ethical, or clinical advice. If legal or other expert advice is required, the services of a competent professional person should be sought.

CPT™® is a registered trademark of the American Medical Association.

Greenbranch Publishing books are available at special quantity discounts for bulk purchases as premiums, fund-raising, or educational use. info@greenbranch.com or (800) 933-3711.

13   8 7 6 5 4 3 2 1

Copyedited, typeset, and printed in the United States of America

PUBLISHER
Nancy Collins

EDITORIAL ASSISTANT
Jennifer Weiss

BOOK DESIGNER
Laura Carter
Carter Publishing Studio

COPYEDITOR
Pat George

Table of Contents

About the Authors viii

Professional Acknowledgments xi

Personal Acknowledgments xii

SECTION I: GETTING STARTED

Introduction 3

Chapter 1: Why Integrate Behavioral Health? 7

Chapter 2: Shared Interprofessional Skills: Language and Collaboration Optimize Operations 15

Chapter 3: What Are Your Needs? 25

Chapter 4: A Menu of Integrated Behavioral Health Options 35

SECTION II: BUSINESS DEVELOPMENT, POLICY, AND OPERATIONS

Chapter 5: Policy 47

Chapter 6: Business Development 55

Chapter 7: Calculating Value and Revenue Cycles 79

Chapter 8: Measuring Your Program's Impact 119

Chapter 9: Hiring 127

Chapter 10: Training 149

Chapter 11: Facilitating the Transition Process to Integrated Care 177

SECTION III: CASE STUDIES, PROFILES, AND EXEMPLARS

Chapter 12: System Initiatives 175

    IMPACT 175

    Colorado Access 177

    Aetna 178

    Cherokee Health Systems 179

    Intermountain Health 180

    Edmonton Southside Primary Care Network 181

    The Piedmont Health Group 182

Glossary 185

About the Authors

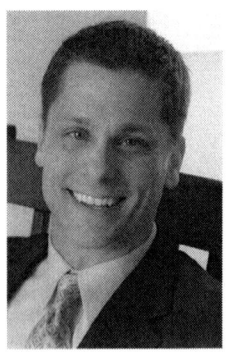

Kent A. Corso, PsyD, BCBA-D, is a licensed clinical health psychologist and board certified behavior analyst. As a veteran of Operation Enduring Freedom, he is a former Air Force officer with 15 years of teaching and training experience in university and medical settings. Dr. Corso currently holds an adjunct assistant professor position in the Department of Family Medicine at the Uniformed Services University of Health Sciences. He leads the primary care behavioral health program for the Military Health System in the Washington, D.C., region, which enrolls more than 137,000 beneficiaries. Dr. Corso is the president of NCR Behavioral Health, a consultation group that assists diverse healthcare delivery systems in the United States and abroad in the development of profitable, cost-saving, quality-enhancing integrated behavioral health programs by leveraging population health principles, cutting-edge practice models, sound business strategies, and high-quality training.

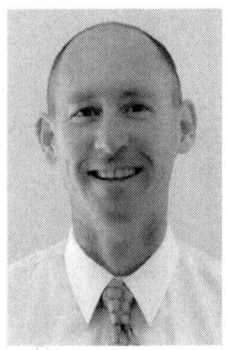

Christopher L. Hunter, PhD, ABPP, graduated from the University of Memphis specializing in behavioral medicine. He is board certified in clinical health psychology and works for the Defense Health Agency as the Department of Defense (DoD) program manager for behavioral health in primary care. As the DoD lead for the last seven years, he has worked to develop policy, secure funding, and oversee the rollout of primary care behavioral health services for 3.3 million Military Health System enrollees. He is a previous chair for the Society of Behavioral Medicine's integrated primary care special interest group and is a Collaborative Family Health Care Association board member. He has extensive experience developing integrated primary care behavioral health services as well as training individuals to work in primary care settings to treat common mental health conditions (e.g., depression), health behavior problems (e.g., tobacco use, obesity) and chronic medical conditions (e.g., diabetes, chronic pain). He is also the lead author on the 2009 book, *Integrated Behavioral Health in Primary Care: Step-by-Step Guidance for Assessment and Intervention* and a co-editor of the 2014 *Handbook of Clinical Psychology in Medical Settings: Evidence-based Assessment and Intervention*.

About the Authors

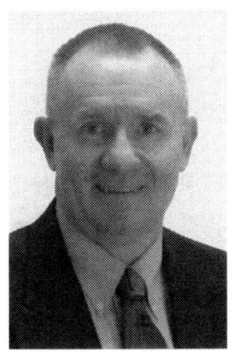

Owen Dahl, MBA, FACHE, CHBC, LSSMBB, has been active in healthcare management for almost 50 years. He received his bachelor's degree from Concordia College, Moorhead, Minnesota, where he was a member of the first graduating class in the hospital administration program. He received his master's degree from the University of Northern Colorado and has done additional study at NOVA Southeastern in Ft. Lauderdale, Florida. He spent more than a decade as a hospital administrator in various facilities in South Dakota. He also served in the United States Air Force and the Army National Guard.

His move to New Orleans in 1983 brought a major career change. He started a practice management and billing company, which grew to manage 65 physicians in 11 different practices. In 1993, he advanced to Fellow in the American College of Health Care Executives with a paper on Total Quality Management and its application to the medical practice. Hurricane Katrina brought about another change that led to his current efforts as an author, consultant, public speaker, and adjunct professor. He has worked with Loyola University in New Orleans, the University of New Orleans, the Louisiana State University School of Medicine, and the University of Houston–Clear Lake on physician practice management programs.

This change came about due to a long-standing passion to seek to improve the delivery of patient care through training and education. He developed the first certification program for the Professional Association of Health Care Office Managers (PAHCOM) and the certification program for the National Society of Certified Health Care Business Consultants (NSCHBC). Currently an independent consultant with an affiliation with the Medical Group Management Association (MGMA), he has developed training programs in various "belt" levels in Lean Six Sigma and the application to today's medical practice. Mr. Dahl is married with three children and two grandchildren. He currently resides in The Woodlands, Texas.

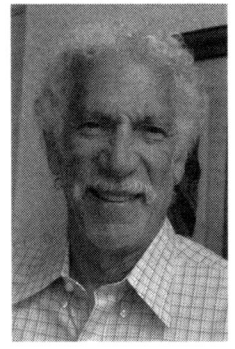

Dr. Gene "Rusty" Kallenberg has been the chief of the Department of Family Medicine and Public Health and vice chair of the Department of Family and Preventive Medicine at the University of California, San Diego (UCSD) since 2001. Previously he was the chief of family medicine and assistant dean for curricular projects at George Washington University (1982–2001). He has been a member of the Collaborative Family Healthcare Association (CFHA) for the past 18 years and is the current president, having served on the board for the past three years and as treasurer. Dr. Kallenberg has overseen the development of integrated behavioral healthcare programs within the PCMH-certified family medicine practices of his Division of Family Medicine (DFM) since 2002. With over 23 part-time trainee, intern, and licensed MFTs and psychologists and psychiatrists, the DFM Collaborative Care Team serves several thousand patients each year. Dr. Kallenberg also is the director of the new UCSD Center for Integrative Medicine, which opened in 2010. Dr. Kallenberg's interests include new models of primary care, mental health/primary care collaboration, integrative medicine and undergraduate/graduate medical education, and competency assessment in the content areas of communication skills, doctor-patient-family relationships, health systems, and professionalism.

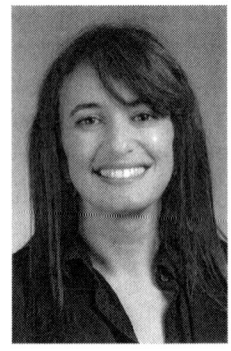

Lesley Manson, PsyD, has spent over a decade providing direct service. Her dedication to behavioral health and integrated care models led her to directing behavioral health programs, providing continuing education to healthcare providers, and developing workshops and trainings for behavioral health and primary care providers to be successful and integral members of healthcare teams. She has advanced experience in continuous quality improvement, behavior change, and standardization and outcome measurement for behavioral health programs integrated into primary care. Dr. Manson has spearheaded multidisciplinary teams for primary care process improvement and population-specific quality improvement and standardization, which has led to improved healthcare outcomes, enhanced quality assurance, increased compliance and patient engagement, and reduced healthcare costs. She was an integral member of teams for the development of electronic medical health records with integrated shared behavioral health focusing on standardization, best practices, and evidence-based techniques. Her history as a healthcare executive has led her to developing national presentations and publications on integration with both clinical and management focus and providing consultation and training for primary care and medical/behavioral organizations in developing and auditing for integrated care sustainability.

Historically, Dr. Manson has been an active member of her local and national professional primary care and behavioral health organizations, serving on numerous boards and receiving recognition. She is a former president of the North Coast Association of Mental Health Professionals in California and was honored with certificate training from the Johnson and Johnson UCLA Health Care Executive Program. She is also a master trainer for the Institute for Health Care Communication and conducts workshops in the area of clinician-patient interaction and communication to meet the Triple Aim. Dr. Manson serves as a clinical assistant professor and director of integrated training initiatives at Arizona State University's Doctor of Behavioral Health Program.

Professional Acknowledgments

This book would not have come to fruition without the consultation, guidance, and support of our colleagues. We would like acknowledge the generous support we received from Jen Funderburk, Anne Dobmeyer, Jeff Reiter, and Jennifer Hodgson.

While working on this project, we learned the term "book widow." One of our spouses coined this phrase. While darkly humorous, this term reminded us of the devotion our spouses offered and sacrifices they made in support of this project. Considering how they managed everything at home and with our families, we are deeply indebted to them.

We thank Nancy Collins and all the staff at Greenbranch, who provided encouragement, flexibility, and vision. This book reflects the collaboration, commitment, and high quality that are the hallmarks of Greenbranch's work.

Personal Acknowledgments

Kent Corso

I am thankful for Meghan Corso, who supported this endeavor and kept our family thriving while we worked on this project. I appreciate the energy and spirit of Stella, Dean, and Siena, who were patient with me and kept me motivated. I am also grateful for the U.S. Air Force, which provided me stellar training and resources in integrated care while I served on active duty. I thank Craig Bryan for his partnership in the clinical research we've conducted together. Lastly, I thank Patti Robinson and Chris Hunter for their training, support, mentorship, and encouragement over the past decade.

Chris Hunter

I would like to thank my wife Christine Hunter for her time and support while engaged in this endeavor. I'd also like to thank my coauthors for their dedication and talent in bringing this work to fruition and all that I have learned from them through this process.

Owen Dahl

I am indeed grateful to my fellow authors for their time, knowledge, and support throughout this project. We, especially me, learned a lot, and I sincerely hope those who read this will continue to work to improve patient care. Special recognition to my wife Noela for her patience and support throughout these many years!

Gene "Rusty" Kallenberg

I thank my colleagues at UCSD Division of Family Medicine/Dept. of Family Medicine and Public Health: William Sieber, PhD, Zephon Lister, MedFT, PhD, and from the USD Marriage and Family Therapy Program: Jo Ellen Patterson, MedFT, PhD, and Todd Edwards, MedFT, PhD.

Lesley Manson

I would like to thank my family for continuing to laugh and appreciate life as a beautiful distraction and reprieve to writing. Further, great appreciation is given to Arizona State University's Doctor of Behavioral Health Program, Open Door Community Health Centers, and the Collaborative Family Healthcare Association. Lastly, I would like to thank my professional colleagues for their continued support and motivation.

SECTION I

Getting Started

Introduction

If you've opened this book, you probably have an idea that integrating behavioral healthcare into primary care is important and consistent with the core principles of a Patient-Centered Medical Home (PCMH) approach to primary healthcare. Or you might have picked up this book while pursuing National Committee for Quality Assurance (NCQA) 2014 PCMH recognition standards[1] which have prompted you to "integrate mental health" services into your system or clinic. Perhaps you were "voluntold" by your boss, board, or other stakeholders to integrate mental health. Or maybe you are simply lucky enough to have stumbled onto this concept and it just makes sense to you.

Regardless of the reason, rest assured the advantages of integrating behavioral health services into primary care, when done well, can lead to better population health outcomes, healthcare cost savings, better healthcare outcomes for general health and mental health compared to traditional primary care, and increased market share for your organization.

TIME IS OF THE ESSENCE

The supporting landscape for integrating behavioral health services into your clinical operation has never been so favorable. In fact, the NCQA's most updated PCMH recognition criteria[1] require the integration of mental health, whereas the 2011 recognition criteria required only "enhanced access" to mental health services. The Patient Protection and Affordable Care Act (PPACA) also brings with it innumerable opportunities to:

- Re-engineer healthcare delivery systems;
- Re-train employees;
- Optimize health outcomes;
- Create new monetization strategies;
- Develop innovative product lines that showcase the organization's value;
- Increase one's market share (i.e., increase the number of patients served by your organization);
- Generate savings/cost offset—True savings is cost management without sacrificing the quality of care. It's doing more with what you have and doing more without spending more money or resources or time. It requires a good understanding of the costs of delivering care effectively and efficiently; and
- Generate revenue—This is generated by contracts, as well as grants, research, direct patient care, and ancillary services. It's also called the "top line."

In short, for the first time in recent history, we have healthcare quality recognition standards, new healthcare laws, healthcare policy, and a primary care service-delivery model that dovetail in an effort to achieve the Triple Aim of improved patient experience, better health outcomes, and lower healthcare costs.[2] This landscape makes integrating mental health services into primary care more likely to be successful than ever before.

HOW DO I USE THIS BOOK?

This book makes for a very poor doorstop, as it is too light. It's too large for a paper-weight. So, your best bet is to use it as a resource for determining what you'll do and how you'll do it. This book offers information that can be immediately applied to:

- Revising your business rules;
- Developing new or revising existing clinical pathways;
- Re-engineering how you provide healthcare to include mental health services;
- Managing the health of your patients; and
- Managing the costs and operational challenges.

Section I provides the context for integrating behavioral health into the medical home. This background conveys critical prerequisite information and enables you to:

- Identify how integrating may benefit you;
- Select goals consistent with your organization's values;
- Envision and manage the operational, cultural, and clinical service delivery paradigm shift that tends to unfold during integration;
- Identify the problems in your organization and patient population for which integration may be part of the solution;
- Use language to facilitate successful integration for your employees and patients; and
- Understand the costs, benefits, and alternatives of various integrated healthcare models.

Section I prepares you with important fundamental concepts and tools relevant to integrated behavioral healthcare (IBH). Its contents help you shape how primary care providers (PCPs) and team members (e.g., nurses, medical assistants) operate, while equipping you to manage the significant changes in how mental health is defined, delivered, and accounted for by all clinical and nonclinical team members.

Section II includes the crux of the business material. While this book is intended to reach our business and healthcare operations colleagues, many of those embarking on integration are chief medical and nursing officers, head primary care providers and nurses, and behavioral health providers who may be responsible for developing the program with sound business principles in mind. As such, our priority for this section was to ensure these tools benefit all these professionals, as well as the diversity of medical home practices—large and small, public and private, pre-integration and post-integration, those dependent on third-party payments entirely, those who are self-sufficient (i.e., HMO), or any blend of these (e.g., FQHC or other grant funding).

You may find some of these tools useful for your organization; other content may be less applicable. Yet, as your integrated program matures, and as health policy, insurance, and other laws continue to evolve over time, some of these payment models may become more relevant to you. Because of the volume of material related to integrating behavioral health into the medical home, the way the field continues to evolve monthly, and the diversity of our intended audience, we have included additional materials and information in the Appendices.

The content we offer will help you:
- Develop a business strategy, business plan, and business case;
- Perform a business case analysis (BCA);
- Estimate a return on investment (ROI);
- Run pro formas (i.e., a method of calculating current or projective fiscal results);
- Manage revenue cycles;
- Hire and train personnel;
- Bill;
- Document;
- Direct workflow; and
- Monitor your program.

We also address methods of analysis and metrics selection so you may conduct program evaluation, program growth or expansion, process improvement, quality assurance, and program sustainment in a manner consistent with your organization's interests and business foci.

Section II also provides suggestions on management, policy development, and operational information, and concludes with in-the-weeds ins and outs of helping your medical home culture adopt behavioral health as part of their "normal" operations.

The last section of the book offers detailed programs of healthcare organizations and systems that have successfully launched IBH in their medical homes. Again, there is diversity among these programs. We included examples of comparable organizations as a snapshot that you could use as a model for developing your own unique services.

We have witnessed small and medium-sized healthcare organizations flounder while attempting IBH. We have witnessed these same struggles in some very large public and private American healthcare organizations. We know from our combined 84 years of integrated care experience that some clear *Do's* and *Don'ts* will help you more rapidly launch your IBH program with fewer errors. To that end, we made deliberate efforts to include only the information you need to make pivotal decisions for your organization, and guidance about the methods needed to be successful. We also provided links for those interested in additional information that might be uniquely applicable to your organization or your phase of implementation.

Implementing these models is as exciting and daunting as the current national challenge of reforming healthcare itself. We hope this book equips you to make rapid, accurate decisions so you are spared the misfortune of failed integration. Whether your organization possesses the ambitious vision or was handed a mandate to initiate an IBH program in your medical home, you deserve a roadmap that helps you achieve this valuable end-goal.

Wait—we almost forgot. You will notice that at the beginning of every chapter we include a summary called "Bottom Line, Up Front." We hope this gives you the most important content, so you can easily understand the take-away messages of each section.

References

1. National Committee for Quality Assurance (NCQA). *Standards and Guidelines for NCQA's Patient-Centered Medical Home (PCMH)*. NCQA, 2014. (Available at http://store.ncqa.org/index.php/2014-pcmh-standards-and-guidelines-epub-single-user.html
2. Institute for Healthcare Improvement (IHI). Initiatives: The IHI Triple Aim Initiative. IHI Web site. http://www.ihi.org/Engage/Initiatives/TripleAim/pages/default.aspx. Accessed April 21, 2015.

CHAPTER 1
Why Integrate Behavioral Health?

BOTTOM LINE, UP FRONT

- Providing primary care and mental healthcare via models we have been using for the past 40 years is no longer tenable. Many indices of American health remain low while costs of our healthcare consistently rise.

- Historically, primary care lacks the mental health component that is critical for improving patients' health.

- Current models for delivering mental health are incomplete and missing components necessary to effectively care for the continuum of mental health difficulties.

- Integrated behavioral healthcare (IBH) creates a "step" in a medical system that has been absent because historically the mental health field specialty has operated in a silo, serving as a "one size fits all" for mental health conditions that patients present to their primary care providers, and providing little to no services for behavioral aspects of general health conditions.

- Mental health care and primary care redesign complement one another. Both warrant new models for workflow; new tools and systems for data collection and documentation; changes in clinic culture, staff, and patient expectations; and fundamental differences in how we deliver care to our patients.

Historically, physical health and mental health have been treated functionally as two separate problem areas. However, in the past 40 years, a growing body of research has demonstrated the connection between physical and mental health. As delineated in Engel's landmark article, to obtain optimal health outcomes, the medical field must attend to the patients' psychological, social, and environmental aspects of their lives as well as their biology.[1]

Following Engel's influential paper, immense research has been conducted on health determinants—those variables that lead to positive or negative health. While some of those health determinants are environmental, economic, cultural, or social, others are specific to the patients themselves. We now know that many of the determinants of poor health in America boil down to simple patient characteristics that are subject to modification without medication or other procedures. Addressing these patient characteristics helps patients achieve better health, often at lower costs to the system. For example, the majority of the variables driving the top 10 causes of death in the United States are attributable to nongenetic and nonbiological factors, and 40% of the factors contributing to premature death in the United States are due to behavioral factors.[2, 3] Patient and family engagement; shared decision making between patient and provider; increased health literacy among patients; improved management of health behaviors (e.g., eating, physical activity, smoking); increased patient engagement and motivation; communication; and trust between patients and providers have all been found to improve illness prevention and chronic disease management, sometimes at lower costs.[4-11]

> **Many of the determinants of poor health in America boil down to simple patient characteristics that are subject to modification without medication or other procedures. Addressing these patient characteristics helps patients achieve better health, often at lower costs to the system.**

Health is no longer as simple as a "physical or mental problem the doctor fixes." Rather, there is growing focus on practical, patient-centered healthcare delivery, where primary care providers (PCPs), behavioral health providers (BHPs), and patients work together to make informed decisions about the best courses of action for optimal physical and mental health. These decisions may include improving medication adherence, adopting a healthier diet, or becoming more physically active. Each of these health-related changes is managed by the BHP in conjunction with the PCP. Studies have shown that this can improve mental health conditions like depression, as well as health conditions like diabetes.[12] Systems that improve information accessibility and sharing, as well as coordination of care across the multiple levels of stepped care, deliver improved outcomes at lower costs through fewer readmissions, fewer unnecessary appointments, less unnecessary emergency department use, and reduced inpatient costs.[13]

Despite the research substantiating how biology, psychological responses, social interaction, and the patient's environment all contribute to the patient's health, many facets of the U.S. healthcare system continue to operate with a reductionist approach, separating physical or general health from mental health. For example, consider that nonpharmacological interventions may be first-line treatments for several of the most common problems seen in primary care (e.g., depression, insomnia, obesity, tension headaches, tobacco use), yet these services often are not available or not ordered by PCPs.[14] In addition, some of the most effective adjunctive treatments for problems like chronic pain, irritable bowel syndrome, and hypertension involve evidence-based psychosocial interventions—those that aren't medications, devices, or medical procedures. In short, this is how behavioral health benefits patients in the medical home.

Yet, the medical system previously had not been primed to incorporate these. Not surprising, the recent past (and sometimes still existing) healthcare payment models reinforced this mindset, along with the years of delayed dissemination and implementation of evidence-based care in training and practice. Even if these barriers are reduced/eliminated, a PCP cannot do it alone.[15] Therefore, integrating appropriately trained BHPs as healthcare team members is important for elevating and extending the care delivery of the entire team. For our purposes, we use the term BHP throughout this book to mean any integrated behavioral health provider in the medical home who can practice independently.

WHY APPROPRIATE BEHAVIORAL HEALTH SERVICES BELONG IN THE MEDICAL HOME

Some may wonder what the benefits are to integrating behavioral health into the medical home. Most of the skeptics we have met are just not well informed, or have had a prior negative experience with integration, that in our estimation, was not a high-quality effort in the first place. The following list helps provide the rationale for integrating behavioral health into the medical home.

- **Reason 1:** Between 30% and 50% of patients referred by a PCP to outpatient mental healthcare never make it to their first appointment.[27, 28] Furthermore, 50% of PCPs report that they can "never, rarely, or sometimes" access high-quality mental health providers to which they can refer their patients.[20] Having integrated BHPs ensures that the team has access to a high-quality provider who can work with the patient and the team on a range of problems and increases the chances that a patient will make that first BHP appointment.
- **Reason 2:** Compared to routine primary care, enhanced primary care behavioral health services deliver superior health outcomes for these conditions: chronic pain, diabetes, obesity, alcohol abuse, tobacco use, depression, generalized anxiety disorder, social anxiety disorder, and panic disorder.[29-41] Positive outcomes also have been found for primary insomnia using integrated BHPs.[42-44] There is often an undetermined wait time for specialty mental health services.
- **Reason 3:** Integrated BHPs typically can provide on-demand same-day services before, after, or in conjunction with appointments with other team members.

- **Reason 4:** Unfortunately, many primary care settings are ill-prepared to manage mental health needs, as reflected by poor detection rates of mental health issues[17, 18] Integrated BHPs can assist with selection and implementation of appropriate screening measures to identify and treat mental health issues that may improve overall health, quality of life, and functioning.
- **Reason 5:** Despite limited psychosocial treatment options[19, 20] between 40% and 60% of patients with psychological disorders are still treated exclusively within primary care.[21, 22, 23] A growing list of studies[24, 25] show that integrated behavioral health in primary care produces superior outcomes to traditional primary care services.
- **Reason 6:** The prevalence of medically unexplained symptoms in primary care range from 20% to 74%.[26] These complaints often are related to adverse childhood experiences (e.g., trauma), current stress, worry or distress of some kind, and therefore, behavioral health interventions may be helpful.
- **Reason 7:** Lower health literacy is consistently associated with increased hospitalizations; increased emergency care use; reduced use of mammography; reduced vaccination against influenza; decreased ability to take medications appropriately; decreased ability to interpret labels and health messages; and, among seniors, poorer overall health status and higher mortality.[16] All of this contributes to higher medical expenses and poorer outcomes. Research on interventions for health literacy find moderate health effects using intensive self-management interventions on health behaviors and disease-management interventions on disease prevalence/severity.[16] Integrated BHPs can develop, deliver, and assist other team members (e.g., nurses, medical assistants) in improving patients' understanding of their health.

Integrating behavioral health services into primary care corrects the historical error in how we understood mental health—as separate from physical health and always as an exceptional need. We have been using a small, specialized, expensive asset (outpatient mental health services) to treat *any* problem that was not considered "physical," even though the problem may have warranted a less-intensive but "nonmedical" treatment that could be efficiently and effectively delivered in primary care.

Integrating behavioral health services into primary care creates an additional level (step) of services that are appropriate for many primary care patients. It avoids underserving (primary care as usual) or overserving (specialty mental health services) the needs of the patient and provides an additional level of care coordination, so those who truly need specialty services can be assisted in getting that care. IBH also facilitates increased care coordination, which advances the goals of the medical home.

This also makes one historical decision tree obsolete: no longer do PCPs ask themselves, "Is this a physical or mental problem?" Rather, they ask, "How can our integrated BHP help my patient with the aspects of care I don't have time to address or that I would prefer to have someone else on my team address?" For more about the benefits of integrated care, consider reviewing the California Mental Health Services Authority resources at www.ibhp.org.

> ***Integrating behavioral health services into primary care corrects the historical error in how we understood mental health—as separate from physical health and always as an exceptional need.***

Throughout this book, we may give the impression that launching an IBH program is as much of a game-changer for traditional primary care as is the implementation of the medical home model itself. IBH is no panacea, but it does have high value, as we have discussed, and is the only *required* integrated specialty for NCQA PCMH recognition. Like primary care, behavioral healthcare is undergoing the most drastic redesign the medical profession has seen in the past half century. The commitment required to launch a medical home is similar to that needed to integrate behavioral health services. Both warrant new models for workflow; new tools and systems for data collection and documentation; changes in clinic culture, staff, and patient expectations; and fundamental differences in how we deliver care to our patients. You really can't have one without the other. As Frank DeGruy, a leader in the field of integrated primary care has stated, " . . . without behavioral health, the medical home fails."

References

1. Engel GL. The need for a new medical model: a challenge for biomedicine. *Science*. 1977: 196 (4286);129-136. http://www.ncbi.nlm.nih.gov/pubmed/847460. Accessed April 12, 2015.
2. McGinnis JM, Williams-Russo P, Knickman JR. The case for more active policy attention to health promotion. *Health Aff*. 2002;21(2):78-93. DOI: 10.1377/hlthaff.21.2.78.
3. Schroeder SA. We can do better: Improving the health of the American people. *N Engl J Med*. 2007;357(12):1221-1228. www.nejm.org. Accessed February 16, 2014.
4. Antecol H, Bedard K. Unhealthy assimilation: Why do immigrants converge to American health status levels? *Demography*. 2006;43(2):337-360. http://www.ncbi.nlm.nih.gov/pubmed/16889132. Accessed November 22, 2014.
5. Bauer AM, Parker MM, Schillinger D, et al. Associations between antidepressant adherence and shared decision making, patient-provider trust and communication among adults with diabetes: Diabetes study of Northern California. *J Gen Intern Med*. 2014;29(8):1139-1147. DOI: 10.1007/s11606-014-2845-6.

6. Berkman ND, Sheridan SL, Donahue KE, et al. Health literacy interventions and outcomes: An updated systematic review. Evidence Report/Technology Assessment No. 199. (Prepared by RTI International–University of North Carolina Evidence-based Practice Center under contract No. 290-2007-10056-I. AHRQ Publication Number 11-E006. Rockville, MD. Agency for Healthcare Research and Quality. March 2011. https://www.pubmedcentral.nih.gov/pubmedhealth/PMH0033249/. Accessed February 16, 2014.
7. Federman AD, Wolf MS, Sofianou A, et al. Self-management behaviors in older adults with asthma: association with health literacy. *J Am Geriatr Soc*. 2014;62(5):872-879. DOI: 10.1111/jgs.12797.
8. Koh HK, Berwick DM, Clancy CM, et al. New federal policy initiatives to boost health literacy can help the nation move beyond the cycle of costly "crisis care." *Health Aff*. 2012; 31(2):1-10. DOI: 10.1377/hlthaf.2011.1169.
9. Lowsky D, Chari R, Hussey PS, Mulcahy A, et al. Flattening the trajectory of healthcare spending: Engage and empower consumers. Report published by The RAND Corporation. 2012. http://www.rand.org/pubs/research_briefs/RB9690z1.html. Accessed April 1, 2015.
10. Schoen C, Osborn R, Doty MM, et al. A survey of primary care physicians in eleven countries, 2009: Perspectives on care, costs, and experiences. *Health Aff*. 2009; 28(6):1171-1183. DOI: 10.1377/hlthaff.28.6.w1171.
11. Thom DH, Hessler D, Willard-Grace R, et al. Does health coaching change patients' trust in their primary care provider? *Patient Educ Couns*. 2014;96(1):136 135-138. DOI: 10.1016/j.pec.2014.03.018.
12. Simon GE, Katon WJ, Lin EH, et al. Cost-effectiveness of systematic depression treatment among people with diabetes mellitus. *Arch Gen Psychiatry*. 2007;64:65-72.
13. Nielsen M, Gibson A, Buelt L, Grundy P, et al. The patient-centered medical home's impact on cost and quality: Annual review of evidence 2013-2014. Patient-Centered Primary Care Collaborative. 2015. https://www.pcpcc.org/download/5499/PCPCC%202015%20Evidence%20Report.pdf. Accessed February 12, 2015.
14. Craven MA & Bland R. Depression in primary care: current and future challenges. *Can J Psychiatry*. 2013 Aug;58(8):442-448. http://search.proquest.com/docview/1429243960/accountid=41151. Accessed January 6, 2015.
15. Corso KA, Dorrance K, LaRochelle J. The physician shortage: a red herring in American healthcare reform. Manuscript submitted to *Military Medicine* as a part of a monograph.
16. Berkman ND, Sheridan SL, Donahue KE, et al. Health Literacy Interventions and Outcomes: An Updated Systematic Review. Evidence Report/Technology Assessment No. 199. (Prepared by RTI International–University of North Carolina Evidence-based Practice Center under contract No. 290-2007-10056-I. AHRQ Publication Number 11-E006. Rockville, MD. Agency for Healthcare Research and Quality. March 2011.
17. Schonfeld WH, Verboncoeur CJ, Fifer SK, et al. The functioning and well-being of patients with unrecognized anxiety disorders and major depressive disorder. *J Affect Disord*. 1997;43(2): 105-119. DOI: 10.1016/S0165-0327(96)01416-4.
18. Williams JW, Noel PH, Cordes JA, Ramirez G et al. Is this patient clinically depressed? *JAMA*. 2002;287(9):1160-1170. DOI: 10.1001/jama.287.9.1160.
19. Kessler RC, Chiu WT, Demler O, Merikangas KR et al. Prevalence, severity, and comorbidity of 12-month DSM-IV disorders in the National Comorbidity Survey Replication. *Arch Gen Psychiatry*. 2005;62(6):617-627. DOI: 10.1001/archpsyc.62.6.617.
20. Trude S, Stoddard JJ. Referral gridlock: primary care physicians and mental health services. *J Gen Internal Med*. 2003;18(6): 442-449. DOI: 10.1046/j.1525-1497.2003.30216.x.
21. Kessler R, Stafford D. Primary care is the de facto mental health system. In Kessler R and Stafford, D. Stafford, eds. In *Collaborative Medicine Case Studies: Evidence in Practice*. New York, NY: Springer Science + Business Media; 2008:9-21.

22. Narrow WE, Regier DA, Rae DS, Manderscheid RW, et al. Use of services by persons with mental and addictive disorders. Findings from the National Institute of Mental Health Epidemiologic Catchment Area Program. *Arch Gen Psychiatry.* 1993;50(2):95-107. DOI: 10.1001/archpsyc.1993.01820140017002.
23. Wang PS, Demler O, Olfson M, et al. Changing profiles of service sectors used for mental health care in the United States. *Am J Psychiatry.* 2006;163(7):1187-1198. DOI: 10.1176/appi.ajp.163.7.1187.
24. Katon W, von Korff M, Lin E, et al. Stepped collaborative care for primary care patients with persistent symptoms of depression: a randomized trial. *Arch Gen Psychiatry.* 1999;56(12):1109-1115. DOI: 10.1001/archpsyc.56.12.1109.
25. Unutzer J, Katon W, Callahan CM, et al. Collaborative care management of late-life depression in the primary care setting: a randomized controlled trial. *JAMA.* 2002;288(22):2836-2845. DOI: 10.1001/jama.288.22.2836.
26. Kroenke K. Physical symptom disorder: a simpler diagnostic category for somatization-spectrum conditions. *J Psychosom Research.* 2006;60(4):335-339. DOI: 10.1016/j.jpsychores.2006.01.022.
27. Fisher L, Ransom DC. Developing a strategy for managing behavioral health care in the context of primary care. Arch Fam Med. 1997;6:324-333. http://triggered.clockss.org/ServeContent?url=http://archfami.ama-assn.org%2Fcgi%2Freprint%2F6%2F4%2F324.pdf. Accessed March 28, 2015.
28. Hoge CW, Auchterlonie JL, Milliken CS. Mental health problems, use of mental health services, and attrition from military service after returning from deployment to Iraq or Afghanistan. *JAMA.* 2006;295(9):1023-1032. DOI: 10.1001/jama.295.9.1023.
29. Butler M, Kane RL, McAlpine D, et al. *Integration of Mental Health/Substance Abuse and Primary Care.* AHRQ Publication No. 09- E003. Rockville, MD. AHRQ. 2008. http://www.ncbi.nlm.nih.gov/books/NBK38632. Accessed December 3, 2014.
30. van Orden M, Hoffman T, Haffmans J, et al. Collaborative mental health care versus care as usual in a primary care setting: a randomized controlled trial. *Psychiatr Serv.* 2009;60(1):74-79. DOI: 10.1176/ps.2009.60.1.74.
31. Gilbody S, Bower P, Fletcher J, et al. Collaborative care for depression: a cumulative meta-analysis and review of longer-term outcomes. *Arch Intern Med.* 2006;166:2314-2321. DOI: 10.1001/archinte.166.21.2314.
32. Williams JW, Gerrity M, Holsinger T, et al. Systematic review of multifaceted interventions to improve depression care. *Gen Hosp Psychiatry.* 2007;29: 91-116. DOI: 10.1016/j.genhosppsych.2006.12.003.
33. Roy-Byrne P, Craske MG, Sullivan G, et al. Delivery of evidence-based treatment for multiple anxiety disorders in primary care: a randomized controlled trial. *JAMA.* 2010;303: 1921-1928. DOI: 10.1001/jama.2010.608.
34. Fiore M, Jaen CR, Baker TB, et al. Treating tobacco use and dependence: 2008 update. *Clinical Practice Guideline.* Rockville, MD: U.S. Department of Health and Human Services, Public Health Service. May 2008. http://www.ahrq.gov/path/tobacco.htm#clinic. Accessed February 4, 2015.
35. Whitlock EP, Polen MR, Green CA, Orleans T, et al. Behavioral counseling interventions in primary care to reduce risky/harmful alcohol use by adults: A summary of the evidence for the U.S. Preventive Services Task Force. *Ann Intern Med.* 2004;140:558-569. DOI: 10.7326/0003-4819-140-7-200404060-00017.
36. Diabetes Prevention Program Research Group. The 10-year cost-effectiveness of lifestyle intervention or metformin for diabetes prevention: An intent-to-treat analysis of the DPP/DPPOS. *Diabetes Care.* 2012;35:723-730. DOI: 10.2337/dc11-1468.
37. Funnell MM, Brown TL, Childs BP, et al. National standards for diabetes self-management education. *Diabetes Care.* 2008;31 Suppl:S97-S104. DOI: 10.2337/dc09-S087.
38. Wadden TA, Volger S, Sarwer DB, et al. A two-year randomized trial of obesity treatment in primary care practice. *NEJM.* 2011;365:1969-1979. DOI: 10.1056/NEJMoa1109220.

39. LeBlanc ES, O'Connor E, Whitlock EP, Patnode CD, et al. Effectiveness of primary care-relevant treatments for obesity in adults: a systematic evidence review for the U.S. Preventive Services Task Force. *Ann Intern Med*. 2011;155:434-447. DOI: 10.7326/0003-4819-155-7-201110040-00006.
40. Ahles TA, Wasson JH, Seville JL, et al. A controlled trial of methods for managing pain in primary care patients with or without co-occurring psychosocial problems. *Ann Fam Med*. 2006; 4(4):341-350. DOI: 10.1370/afm.527.
41. Dobscha SK, Corson K, Perrin NA, et al. Collaborative care for chronic pain in primary care: a cluster randomized trial. *JAMA*. 2009;301(12):1242-1252. DOI: 10.1001/jama.2009.377.
42. Edinger JD, Sampson WS. A primary care" friendly" cognitive behavioral insomnia therapy. *Sleep*. 2003;26(2):177-184. http://www.researchgate.net/profile/William_Sampson2/publication/1816262_A_primary_care_friendly_cognitive_behavioral_insomnia_therapy/links/0fcfd50ba6bddb2c24000000.pdf. Accessed September 8, 2015.
43. Goodie JL, Isler WC, Hunter C, et al. Using behavioral health consultants to treat insomnia in primary care: a clinical case series. *J Clin Psychol*. 2010;65(3):294-304. DOI: 10.1002/jclp.20548.
44. Sadock E, Auerbach SM, Rybarczyk B, et al. Evaluation of integrated psychological services in a university-based primary care clinic. *J Clin Psychol Med Settings*. 2014;21(1):19-32. DOI: 10.1007/s10880-013-9378-8.

CHAPTER 2

Shared Interprofessional Skills: Language and Collaboration Optimize Operations

BOTTOM LINE, UP FRONT

- Deliberately select interprofessional language for broad use and then standardize this language, as this optimizes a team's ability to function and increases the *patient-centeredness* of your services.

- Use such language regularly up and down your organization's ladder and across your system to help your integrated culture develop. Standardized language supports customer service (and therefore healthcare quality) because patients will develop a clear understanding of who all of their medical providers are and *how* these providers benefit them.

- Train your staff on shared interprofessional collaboration skills. The medical model historically trains personnel to function in a hierarchy, not as a team.

- When your staff uses standardized language and well-defined interprofessional collaborative skills, patients benefit and, consequently, your organization does, too.

At the department or clinic levels, standardizing language and creating well-defined roles helps individual team members understand their own place within the larger team, and understand and interact with all other team members more effectively. This concept is so important that a growing number of organizations have published guidance on this subject. Many, including the Agency for Healthcare Research and Quality (AHRQ), have advocated shared language in integrated care settings as an important way to improve healthcare quality.[1-4] The remainder of this section provides tools for creating shared interprofessional language and collaboration skills in your organization, including a few sources whose models you may choose to use or adapt to meet your medical home needs.

LANGUAGE

We all use similar language in the medical field; but with different specialties increasingly coming together to deliver team-based care, it is important to have a shared interprofessional language to ensure optimized team communication and collaboration. Devising a shared interprofessional language is important. It will facilitate effective communication in this rapidly evolving area of the field for healthcare policy makers; business development, finance, and accounting personnel; researchers and program evaluators; clinicians; medical groups; healthcare plans; purchasers of healthcare plans; and patients and families.[1]

For our purposes, we use the words *program, product line,* and *service* interchangeably, knowing that these have different nuances conceptually and operationally. We also acknowledge that there is a movement afoot to use the words primary care clinician instead of primary care provider. While we value the rationale behind this, in order to use terms which are familiar to a broad audience, we used primary care provider [PCP] throughout this book.) We also use the word payer throughout this book even thought that usually refers to the patient, while payor usually refers to the third party who reimburses health care costs. For simplicity we have used payer to signify both.

Key interprofessional language terms in this book are taken from the *Lexicon for Mental Health and Primary Care Integration*,[1, 4] which provides a comprehensive review of this language. If you are interested in implementing a few key terms for shared interprofessional language as you launch integrated behavioral healthcare (IBH), consult this resource first (Figure 2.1).

Operationally defined interprofessional terms:

Integrated care—tightly integrated, onsite teamwork with unified care plans as a standard approach to care. It connotes organizational integration involving social and other services. It includes integrated treatments, program structures, systems of programs, and payments.[1, 4]

Behavioral healthcare—an umbrella category for provider services focused on behaviors (emotions and thoughts) that affect any health or mental health condition. In this sense, it is broader than mental health and substance abuse. It also includes educating and motivating patients, helping them set goals, helping them adhere to any provider's treatment plan, and treating symptoms of any health or mental health condition by helping patients develop healthier behaviors, habits, routines, and thoughts.[1] This may also involve assisting the patient in understanding, monitoring, and managing his/her emotions. The literature also refers to this as mind/body medicine and mental medicine, and it is sometimes included in the list of treatments under "complementary and alternative medicines" (CAMS). Table 2.1 lists all the conditions for which the evidence-based literature supports

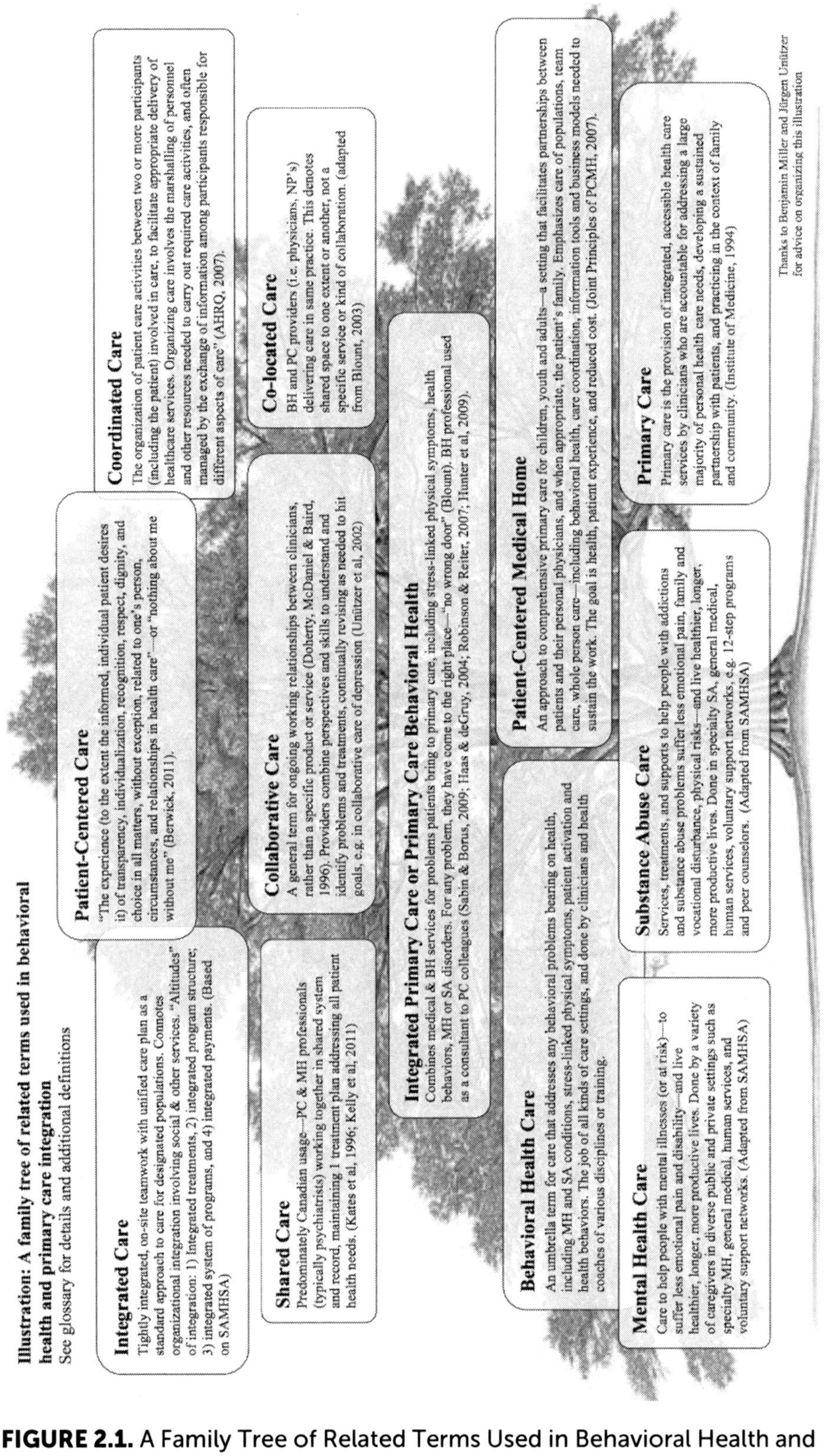

Illustration: A family tree of related terms used in behavioral health and primary care integration
See glossary for details and additional definitions

Integrated Care
Tightly integrated, on-site teamwork with unified care plan as a standard approach to care for designated populations. Connotes organizational integration involving social & other services. "Altitudes" of integration: 1) Integrated treatments, 2) integrated program structure; 3) integrated system of programs, and 4) integrated payments. (Based on SAMHSA)

Shared Care
Predominantly Canadian usage—PC & MH professionals (typically psychiatrists) working together in shared system and record, maintaining 1 treatment plan addressing all patient health needs. (Kates et al, 1996; Kelly et al, 2011)

Patient-Centered Care
"The experience (to the extent the informed, individual patient desires it) of transparency, individualization, recognition, respect, dignity, and choice in all matters, without exception, related to one's person, circumstances, and relationships in health care" — or "nothing about me without me" (Berwick, 2011).

Collaborative Care
A general term for ongoing working relationships between clinicians, rather than a specific product or service (Doherty, McDaniel & Baird, 1996). Providers combine perspectives and skills to understand and identify problems and treatments, continually revising as needed to hit goals, e.g. in collaborative care of depression (Unützer et al, 2002)

Integrated Primary Care or Primary Care Behavioral Health
Combines medical & BH services for problems patients bring to primary care, including stress-linked physical symptoms, health behaviors, MH or SA disorders. For any problem, they have come to the right place—"no wrong door" (Blount). BH professional used as a consultant to PC colleagues (Sabin & Borus, 2009; Haas & deGruy, 2004; Robinson & Reiter, 2007; Hunter et al, 2009).

Behavioral Health Care
An umbrella term for care that addresses any behavioral problems bearing on health, including MH and SA conditions, stress-linked physical symptoms, patient activation and health behaviors. The job of all kinds of care settings, and done by clinicians and health coaches of various disciplines or training.

Mental Health Care
Care to help people with mental illnesses (or at risk)—to suffer less emotional pain and disability—and live healthier, longer, more productive lives. Done by a variety of caregivers in diverse public and private settings such as specialty MH, general medical, human services, and voluntary support networks. (Adapted from SAMHSA)

Coordinated Care
The organization of patient care activities between two or more participants (including the patient) involved in care, to facilitate appropriate delivery of healthcare services. Organizing care involves the marshalling of personnel and other resources needed to carry out required care activities, and often managed by the exchange of information among participants responsible for different aspects of care" (AHRQ, 2007).

Co-located Care
BH and PC providers (i.e. physicians, NP's) delivering care in same practice. This denotes shared space to one extent or another, not a specific service or kind of collaboration. (adapted from Blount, 2003)

Patient-Centered Medical Home
An approach to comprehensive primary care for children, youth and adults—a setting that facilitates partnerships between patients and their personal physicians, and when appropriate, the patient's family. Emphasizes care of populations, team care, whole person care—including behavioral health, care coordination, information tools and business models needed to sustain the work. The goal is health, patient experience, and reduced cost. (Joint Principles of PCMH, 2007).

Substance Abuse Care
Services, treatments, and supports to help people with addictions and substance abuse problems suffer less emotional pain, family and vocational disturbance, physical risks—and live healthier, longer, more productive lives. Done in specialty SA, general medical, human services, voluntary support networks, e.g. 12-step programs and peer counselors. (Adapted from SAMHSA)

Primary Care
Primary care is the provision of integrated, accessible health care services by clinicians who are accountable for addressing a large majority of personal health care needs, developing a sustained partnership with patients, and practicing in the context of family and community. (Institute of Medicine, 1994)

Thanks to Benjamin Miller and Jürgen Unützer for advice on organizing this illustration

FIGURE 2.1. A Family Tree of Related Terms Used in Behavioral Health and Primary Care Integration

TABLE 2.1. Examples of Conditions Commonly Treated by Integrated Behavioral Health Professionals

Insomnia	Weight Loss	Depression
Chronic Pain	Tobacco Cessation	Anxiety
Diabetes	Sexual Dysfunction	Suicidal Ideation
Hypertension	Grief	Situational Stress

nonpharmacological interventions as the first-line treatment or as an adjunctive treatment for mental and general health conditions.

Behavioral health also involves prevention, outreach, educational, health promotions, and population health activities for all patients enrolled in the medical home. Keep these details in mind when you develop your business plan in Section II, as the prevalence of these conditions among your patient population, or their needs for education and treatment, may influence your business plan for IBH.

Integrated behavioral healthcare (IBH)—combines the two preceding terms. It is integrated care, as we have described, but the type of services that are integrated involve behavioral healthcare as defined above.

Behavioral health provider (BHP)—refers to any licensed independent practitioner you integrate into your medical home in an integrated behavioral healthcare role; typically, this term excludes nonlicensed independent practitioners who provide IBH.

Mental healthcare—refers to services that *exclusively* help people with mental illnesses (or are at risk for mental illness).[1, 4] In this book, we use the term "specialty mental healthcare" to refer to these services, meaning outpatient mental health services.

Patient-centered care—the patient experience of transparent, individualized, recognized, respected, dignified, and elected care related to one's own circumstances and relationships.[5]

Patient-Centered Medical Home (PCMH)—an approach to comprehensive primary care for children, youth, and adults. PCMH facilitates partnerships between patients and their personal physicians, and when appropriate, their family; emphasis is on caring for populations, team-based care, and holistic care.[1, 6] PCMH aims to improve the quality, cost, accessibility, and efficiency of primary care by increasing the availability of appointments and by separating members of the clinic into smaller multidisciplinary teams consisting of a few primary care providers, nurses, and other paraprofessionals.

The PCMH takes daily actions to predict and proactively address scheduling, billing, and staffing problems and encourages all personnel within the clinic to practice at the peak of their professional training and scope of practice. The PCMH additionally integrates a range of medical and health specialties into the clinic's teams in order to keep patients more closely tied to their "home" clinic. These additional specialists might include nutritional medicine, health promotions, mental health (traditional specialty mental health, also called co-located specialty mental health), alternative and complementary medicine, physical medicine, and pharmacy.[7,8]

As you move forward, regardless of the terms you use, make sure they are operationally defined in a way that makes sense for your setting. Ensure the nonclinical staff and leadership understand these new terms and use them correctly. It can be embarrassing when a healthcare executive fails to accurately describe product lines or services to stakeholders. It is equally unhelpful and can have a negative effect on care coordination or patient experience when a clinical or nonclinical staff member confuses patients by using unfamiliar terms or the same terms the rest of the team is using, but with a different implied meaning.

INTERPROFESSIONAL COLLABORATION SKILLS

Effective medical home service delivery requires professionals to communicate and collaborate while coordinating patient care in teams versus hierarchies. Frequently, those responsible for launching medical homes carry the responsibility of ensuring all staff possess these team-based skills. It sounds silly, "doctors and nurses not knowing how to work as teams . . ." but despite the fact that a medical home hallmark is team-based care, there is a paucity of training for care team staff on these skills.

Traditional care delivery models taught in medical, nursing, and graduate school do not address team intervention skills. If you doubt the relevance of this occupational shift, simply interview all your medical assistants, nurses, and primary care providers (PCPs) and ask them the following "Yes/No" questions:

1) Do you generally practice differently today than the way you did 5–10 years ago in the same job?
2) Is it easy to balance the new demands of the medical home model with the amount of time and resources you have?
3) Are you using the highest level of skills your license and certifications allow?
4) Are you as efficient as you could possibly be each day?
5) Do patients understand the tenets of the medical home model the way you do?
6) Could you describe every type of professional in your medical home and the unique role each plays, if a patient asked?

If the answers to any of these questions is "no," your staff would benefit from *at least some* initial training in interprofessional collaboration skills. Problems in these areas can impede optimal medical home team functioning. This is why there is such a widespread movement for interprofessional language and training for team-based care.

TABLE 2.2. Core Competencies for Interprofessional Collaborative Practice: Specific Interprofessional Communication Competencies

Interprofessional Communication Competency	Competency Number	Integrated Healthcare Redesign	Integrated Team-Based Care Planning
Provide effective communication tools and techniques, including information systems and communication technologies to facilitate discussions and interactions that enhance team function.	CC1	Creation of electronic health records (EHR) with interprofessional documentation, review, and communication exchange. Data pulling capabilities for analysis and review.	Training and use of EHR documentation to create integrated care paths and integrated plans of care with interactive review of goals and documentation by the care team.
Organize and communicate information with patients, families, and healthcare team members in a form that is understandable, avoiding discipline-specific terminology when possible.	CC2	Utilize health literacy and numeracy tools. Ensure verbal and written communication is provided at an appropriate language level. Practice identifying laymen verbiage to replace discipline-specific terminology. Create scripts.	Create scripts for team-based care and ensure laymen language is used throughout the care team, paired with terminology needed to ensure clarity of communication.
Express one's knowledge and opinions to team members involved in patient care with confidence, clarity, and respect, working to ensure common understanding of information and treatment and care decisions.	CC3	Ensure the patient's own words related to progress and goals are documented.	Team-based care is aligned in the integrated plan of care, acknowledging use of the patient's own words as well as care team members' roles and activity on the care plan.
Listen actively and encourage ideas and opinions of other team members.	CC4	Practice reflective listening techniques with patients; ensure clarity in communication and ask for feedback on interpretation.	Establish a care team meeting monthly to review cases needed; identify a care team staffing leader to operationalize the group and ensure facilitation of communication by each member.

Continued on next page

Interprofessional Communication Competency	Competency Number	Integrated Healthcare Redesign	Integrated Team-Based Care Planning
Give timely, sensitive, instructive feedback to others about their performance on the team, responding respectfully as a team member to feedback from others.	CC5	Train interprofessional care teams for succinct and relevant communication related to patient outcomes, care needs, and role development; train teams on interprofessional laws and ethical standards; train teams on succinct delivery of shared language role descriptions within the care team.	Practice team-based care delivery with succinct communication within the care team as well as with the patient and his or her family to facilitate feedback and use of reflective listening.
Use respectful language appropriate for a given difficult situation, crucial conversation, or interprofessional conflict.	CC6	Ensure shared language is identified for communication of legal, ethical, and professional dilemmas; train for shared language in conflict resolution; provide empathy training.	Ensure shared language.
Recognize how one's own uniqueness, including experience level, expertise, culture, power, and hierarchy within the healthcare team, contributes to effective communication, conflict resolution, and positive interprofessional working relationships.	CC7	Ensure each member of the care team succinctly utilizes shared language to communicate his or her role, value, and scope of practice. Consider training on literacy-level shared communication and motivational interviewing techniques.	Ensure language related to role, value, and scope of practice is within literacy level for clear understanding by each member of the care team, patient, and his or her family.
Communicate consistently the importance of teamwork in patient-centered and community-focused care.	CC8	Ensure staffing, meetings, and culture of clinic and organization are reflective of team-based and interprofessional care; facilitate effective communication and team member inclusion.	Use shared language with patients and their families about the value of integrated care and team-based healthcare. Utilize shared language to discuss patient-centered and community-focused care.

Although we present more training resources in Chapter 9, an excellent resource for this topic is the "Core Competencies for Interprofessional Collaborative Practice: Specific Interprofessional Communication Competencies." We list some of the contents of this document in Table 2.2. The core competencies were developed in 2011 by the American Association of Colleges of Nursing, Association of Colleges of Osteopathic Medicine, American Association Colleges of Pharmacy Education, Association of American Medical Colleges, and Association of Schools of Public Health.[9]

One note about training your staff on shared interprofessional language and collaborative practice: Consider leveraging your behavioral health professionals and medical home leaders to help train the staff. Such an action illustrates the sort of collaboration you expect in your medical home. As staff members develop these skills, you will likely benefit from a more patient-centered culture and more efficient workflow.

One simple way to start, as suggested by the Institute for Patient and Family Centered Care, is by having every professional in your organization use a standard introduction at the beginning of all patient encounters (for secure messaging, by telephone and in person) describing who they are and how they fit into your care team. While this sounds cumbersome, particularly in smaller organizations, this 20- to 30-second introduction improves customer service and the patient-centeredness of your care.

When patients understand what the integrated behavioral health provider, integrated pharmacist, dietician, diabetes nurse educator, team nurse, and PCP each do, they know whom to contact for their various needs. This aligns your patients' expectations with yours and shares your vision with patients for how care will be delivered per your medical home.

References

1. Peek CJ, National Integration Academy Council. *Lexicon for Mental Health and Primary Care Integration: Concepts and Definitions Developed by Expert Consensus.* AHRQ Publication No.13-IP001-EF. Rockville, MD: Agency for Healthcare Research and Quality; 2013. Available at: http://integrationacademy.ahrq.gov/sites/default/files/Lexicon.pdf.
2. Center for Advancing Health. *A New Definition of Patient Engagement: What Is Engagement and Why Is It Important?* Washington, DC: Center for Advancing Health; 2010. www.cfah.org. Downloaded January 16, 2015.
3. Collins C, Hewson, DL, Munger R, Wade T. *Evolving Models of Behavioral Health Integration in Primary Care.* New York, NY: Milbank Memorial Fund; 2010. Available at: http://www.milbank.org/uploads/documents/10430EvolvingCare/10430EvolvingCare.html
4. SAMHSA-HRSA Center for Integrated Health Solutions Web sites: http://www.integration.samhsa.gov; http://www.integration.samhsa.gov/resource/standard-framework-for-levels-of-integrated-healthcare.
5. Berwick D. What "patient-centered" should mean: Confessions of an extremist. *Health Aff.* 28(4):560-562. DOI: 10.1377/hlthaff.28.4.w555.

6. Patient-Centered Primary Care Collaborative. *Joint Principles of Patient-Centered Medical Home.* 2007. www.pcpcc.net. Accessed September 8, 2015.
7. Ferrante JM, Balasubramanian B, Hudson SV, Crabtree BF. Principles of the patient-centered medical home and preventive services. *Ann Fam Med.* 2010;8:108-116. DOI: 10.1370/afm.1080.
8. Rittenhouse DR, Shortell SM. The Patient-Centered Medical Home: will it stand the test of health reform? *JAMA.* 2009;301(19): 2038-2040. DOI:10.1001/jama.2009.691.
9. Interprofessional Education Collaborative Expert Panel. *Core Competencies for Interprofessional Collaborative Practice: Report of an Expert Panel.* Washington D.C.: Interprofessional Education Collaborative; 2011. http://www.aacn.nche.edu/education-resources/ipecreport.pdf. Accessed April 3, 2015.

CHAPTER 3
What Are Your Needs?

> **BOTTOM LINE, UP FRONT**
> - Implementing integrated behavioral healthcare (IBH), like the medical home, involves significant change.
> - Complete the checklist and staff surveys in this chapter. They will save you time, money, and resources that might otherwise be wasted without taking these preparatory steps.
> - Don't skip it.
> - ... no really, don't skip it

Even with the right training and interest in assessing and treating mental health conditions in primary care, primary care providers (PCPs) often refer patients with these problems outside of the clinic because of their limited time or other financial or organizational factors. This is why many organizations use the IBH service specifically to augment what the rest of the medical home team is doing. Accordingly, your organization's needs and reasons for integrating likely will drive the model you select. The following sections list important areas of consideration, including your clinic philosophy, patient population, staff members' needs, and your healthcare goals.

ASSESSING YOUR NEEDS

Mental and physical healthcare historically have been separated from one another. Moreover, unhelpful historic conceptualizations and misunderstandings of mental health and behavioral health (none of which apply to you, of course, since you've fully digested the content of Chapters 1 and 2) may render some medical practices struggling with how to best "house" behavioral health under one roof. In many cases, the lead PCPs and nurses in the clinic will report that they don't know how to help the BHP get up and running because they are unfamiliar with the needs of these professionals.

This is relevant to assessing your needs, because your BHPs need what your PCPs need, not in terms of equipment, but in terms of leadership support, inclusion in all clinic issues and priorities, and administrative support at the clinical level. Consider treating your BHP as an essential component of the care you provide in primary care, and no different than one of your PCPs.

Below is a preparation checklist. Think of it as a warm-up for your business plan. Initially, consider answering these questions without conducting extensive research on your clinic (e.g., finances, patient population). Also consider photocopying this list and having your clinical, non-clinical, and management staff complete it as a way to help assess their interest in and receptiveness to integration. If they are not receptive or don't see the relevance, it will be important for you to help them learn why integrated behavioral health services are important to patients, and will help the team practice more effectively and efficiently attain its goals.

> *Consider treating your BHP as an essential component of the care you provide in primary care, and no different than one of your PCPs.*

System change is often difficult. Feedback can reveal changes your staff would welcome, which can serve as initial targets for change. Consider reviewing this list again when conducting your business case analyses (BCAs), at which point you should probably collect more in-depth data about your organization (See Chapters 6 and 7).

PROPOSING THE INITIATIVE TO YOUR PCPS

One way to effectively trigger a revolt among your PCP staff is to mandate practice processes, models, or tools without securing any buy-in from them. Therefore, during these planning stages (before conducting BCAs), consider sampling your PCPs' attitudes toward the behavioral health issues they face. First, you should define the important terms for your staff using standard interprofessional language (See Chapter 2) so your polling results accurately reflect commonly defined problems, clinical and workflow expectations, and your PCPs' beliefs about the prospect of integrating behavioral health.

Most PCPs today have had some training in mental health issues commonly seen in primary care, but their views of the relative importance of these issues versus medical issues, and whether they are "their business" can vary markedly. PCPs' comfort level in dealing with a patient's emotional disclosure can also vary. If they are not comfortable handling patient expressions of emotion, do not feel at ease assessing such problems, or don't know how to assist patients including how/where/when to refer these patients for additional help, they likely will avoid mental health issues. Some may simply find it easier to avoid opening

PREPARATION CHECKLIST

- [ ] Who would you like to use this service?
  - What percent of your patient population do you intend to reach with this service?
  - Are you looking to serve a specific population (e.g., children and adolescents, geriatric patients, patients with substance abuse habits, etc.)?
  - Are you interested in better disease management specifically for one disorder (e.g., depression, diabetes, chronic pain)?
  - Is your desire to help as many patients in your population as you can?
- [ ] What staffing, IT, space, and other resources do you already have to help implement this program?
- [ ] What financial resources can you identify?
- [ ] What is your desired timeline for implementation?
- [ ] What is your desired timeline for gaining a return on investment (ROI)?
- [ ] What are your related accreditation or other regulatory goals and pressures?
- [ ] What is the motivation and "buy-in" among your leadership to developing integrated behavioral healthcare?
- [ ] How high is your clinical staff's motivation to address mental health needs?
- [ ] What is your staff's current understanding of mental health? Consider sharing Figure 2.1 with your staff, as mental health covers a wide range of clinical areas, from patient motivation for health behavior change, to health goal setting, mental health treatment, and managing acute and chronic conditions through nonpharmacological means.
- [ ] What resources do you have to manage this paradigm shift as you launch?
- [ ] How ready is your staff to tackle new and exciting ways to deliver healthcare?
- [ ] What are the needs and values of your patients (e.g., low health literacy, expectations for delivery of healthcare)?
- [ ] What are your clinical staff members' assets and challenges with regard to delivering care via team-based methods, communication, exploring patients' values and preferences, and enabling patients to follow through with often-difficult mental and behavioral health changes needed to maintain or improve health?
- [ ] How are you doing on Healthcare Effectiveness Data and Information Set (HEDIS) metrics related to diabetes, depression, and pain care for adults? What about your HEDIS metrics for children and adolescents?
- [ ] What are your most costly chronic diseases?
- [ ] How much is patient nonadherence costing you financially? How much damage is it doing in preventing positive health in your patient population? To what extent does it inconvenience your practice?
- [ ] Is high utilization a problem (e.g., increasing overall cost of care, decreasing clinic efficiency or access)? How does this affect your practice?
- [ ] How does your staff see behavioral health services being best integrated into what your medical home already offers?
- [ ] What aspects of your patients' health would receive more attention if you had an immediately accessible behavioral health resource daily?

Pandora's Box. Still, there is much evidence that PCPs miss or ignore psychosocial variables patients reveal during medical appointments—much of which is emotional content, body language, or other direct attempts to bring up mental issues during visits.[1-3]

One way to secure early buy-in from these stakeholders is by eliciting their thoughts and opinions through survey questionnaires like the one in Table 3.1. Collecting this information and providing feedback about the results, including the opportunity to discuss the results, can help steer your organization toward models of integrated behavioral healthcare the PCPs will appreciate and use. This process can facilitate a common understanding across the medical and business staff (e.g., managers, administrators) that behavioral healthcare issues *are indeed* important in their own right, that they do affect patients' overall health, that they are "PCPs' business," and that PCPs can learn to handle them more efficiently and effectively with the assistance of IBH services. The survey included in Table 3.1 may also be used as a pre-post measure to compare scores before and sometime after you launch IBH.

Keep in mind that the maturity of your medical home may partially drive your PCPs' response to this questionnaire. So if your medical home is struggling to conduct huddles, implement team-based care, scrub schedules in advance, use e-mail and phone methods to conduct some care, facilitate all staff to operate at the peak of their relative specialty, optimize access, achieve high customer satisfaction metrics (or even collect them at all), and strive for the Triple Aim, they may be overwhelmed or uninformed about IBH and therefore favor a co-located specialty mental health model in which specialty mental health services are located inside the clinic for their use.

We discuss several models of integrated behavioral health service delivery in the following chapter, but for now, know that the maturity of your medical home can shape your PCPs' interest in IBH.

PREPARE, PLAN, PREPARE, PLAN

Preparing prior to program initiation, securing buy-in from all stakeholders, anticipating obstacles, and developing solutions in advance can help avoid program failures and staff and patient dissatisfaction with your new services. DO NOT simply read the primary literature about integrated care, or hire a BHP to do so, and then attempt to launch your program. This is like reading your car's owner's manual and then attempting to build a similar car by yourself. In 2014, The RAND Corporation published a report summarizing their study of 56 integrated care programs that were grant-funded by the Substance Abuse and Mental Health Services Administration (SAMHSA). The outcomes were not as impressive as they could have been. The report concluded that not fully developing or implementing

Chapter 3—What Are Your Needs?

TABLE 3.1. Provider Survey

Name (optional): _____ Date: _____ Age: _____ Sex: M F
Terminal degree you possess (M.D., Ph.D., RN, etc.) _____ Date Conferred _____
Specialty (e.g., Family Medicine, Pediatrics, Internal Medicine) _____
Type of clinic / practice: _____ Name of clinic: _____
State of practice: _____ Average number of patients you see per week: _____

Please rate your agreement with the following statements:

strongly disagree	somewhat disagree	slightly disagree	slightly agree	moderately agree	strongly agree
1	2	3	4	5	6

1		Mental health problems are as important to identify and treat as general health problems.
2		My residency program had a strong commitment to mental health training.
3		I have good diagnostic skills in the area of mental health.
4		If a need is identified, I prefer to receive consultation with a behavioral health professional rather than automatically refer a patient to treatment.
5		I have good mental health counseling skills.
6		It is difficult to reach mental health colleagues for an informal consultation.
7		I actively look for psychiatric disorders in my patient population.
8		I have been satisfied with the amount of contact I have with behavioral health providers regarding the care of my patients.
9		I'm uncomfortable telling a patient I made a psychiatric diagnosis and am recommending treatment.
10		Behavioral health professionals can be especially useful in helping a patient change a health behavior (e.g., improve diet, increase adherence to treatment, child mental management).
11		Patients' physical health and recovery from illness are influenced significantly by their emotional health and the level of social support available to them.
12		Treatment of mental health problems has a much lower rate of success than most medical problems.
13		There are areas in working with psychiatric problems for which I would like to have more background and skills.
14		My current practice setting has a strong commitment to using patients' family members as a resource in patient care.
15		It is important to ask my patients about their family relationships.
16		My psychopharmacology skills are excellent.
17		I understand the effects of family relationships on health.
18		I am satisfied with the current referral process for behavioral health services.
19		Minor psychiatric symptoms take up too much of my time.
20		I understand the effects of illness on family relationships.
21		Consulting with or including behavioral health professionals in joint treatment planning is often unnecessary.

22		I have benefited from consultations with mental health professionals.
23		I know how to easily contact a behavioral health professional for a patient consultation.
24		I provide brief psychosocial interventions myself.
25		Incorporating services of behavioral health experts in a patients' care is often vital.
26		My patients have easy access to a behavioral medicine (i.e., pain management, sleep hygiene, medication adherence) or mental health (e.g., family therapy) professional.
27		I frequently use behavioral medicine specialists to support patient lifestyle change (i.e., smoking, weight loss).
28		Part of the role of a PCP is to identify behavioral health problems.
29		Part of the role of a PCP is to treat behavioral health problems.
30		Part of the role of a PCP is to involve behavioral health colleagues in treating mental or general health problems.

The following questions ask for percentages between 0% and 100%.

31		What % of your patients present with some mental health or behavioral medicine needs?
31b		For what % of these patients do you attempt to involve a mental health or behavioral medicine professional?
31c		Of these patients, what % keep at least one appointment with this professional?
31d		For what % of these patients do you exchange their information with this professional?
31e		For what % of these patients are you personally acquainted with this professional?
31f		Of these patients, for what % do you meet with the professional to coordinate treatment planning?

For which of these patient conditions/symptoms are behavioral health colleagues most likely to be helpful?

	Depression		Anxiety		Eating disorders
	Bipolar disorder		Psychotic symptoms		Sleep disorders
	Dementia		Social difficulties		Weight management
	Chronic pain		Smoking cessation		Marital/family problems
	Psychiatric diagnostic clarification		Medication/treatment adherence		
	Substance abuse counseling		Adjustment to new medical diagnosis		

Please estimate the number of times over the past year you have made referrals to behavioral health colleagues for each of the following conditions/symptoms.

	Depression		Anxiety		Eating disorders
	Bipolar disorder		Psychotic symptoms		Sleep disorders
	Dementia		Social difficulties		Weight management
	Chronic pain		Smoking cessation		Marital/family problems

	Psychiatric diagnosis clarification		Medication/treatment adherence		
	Substance abuse counseling		Adjustment to new medical diagnosis		

When my patients require behavioral health services, I typically refer them to a professional:
- ☐ Who is located in another group/facility/organization.
- ☐ Who is a member of my group/organization but is *not* located in my office suite.
- ☐ Who is located right in my office suite *AND*:
- ☐ We have separate office systems (e.g. charts, administrative staff).
- ☐ We share office systems.

When I communicate with a behavioral health provider, I most often use:
☐ e-mail   ☐ letters   ☐ phone   ☐ face-to-face meetings

How satisfied are you with your patients' **access** to behavioral health services?

1	2	3	4	5	6	7	8	9	10
extremely dissatisfied									extremely satisfied

How satisfied are you with the **quality** of behavioral health services your patients receive?

1	2	3	4	5	6	7	8	9	10
extremely dissatisfied									extremely satisfied

What barriers do you face when arranging for patients to receive behavioral healthcare?

Thank you for your valuable time in completing this survey

Adapted with permission from Sieber, Kallenberg, and Patterson (unpublished scale)

---

a clear model and program (i.e., not implementing a specific, structured, and well-developed model), and low patient program use were among the primary reasons limiting success. Additional publications have argued that these shortcomings need to be improved for future integration programs to maximize success.[4, 5]

Consider reviewing the resources posted on the Web site for the Patient-Centered Primary Care Collaborative (PCPCC): www.pcpcc.org/publications. They provide information about patient-centered care, optimizing your medical home, behavioral health in pediatrics, and the various issues related to IBH services. They may be especially helpful for gaining stakeholder buy-in and averting problems associated with clinical staff not being ready or receptive to IBH.

> ***DO NOT simply read the primary literature about integrated care, or hire a BHP to do so, and then attempt to launch your program. This is like reading your car's owner's manual and then attempting to build a similar car by yourself.***

While it is logical for primary care organizations to seek integration through partnership with local mental health organizations, this venture is exceedingly difficult. At the ground level, most of these mental health professionals will have no experience with integrated care. That's to say, they commonly operate independently—not as part of a team; with little interest, experience, or knowledge in the medical aspects of patients; and with limited understanding of the primary care culture and the medical home model. Some would say that historically, specialty mental health providers have conducted care in a way that inadvertently excludes the patient's primary care team. Also, the majority of mental health providers have little-to-no training in the highly specific core skills required to deliver IBH models.

Simply contracting services out to a mental health organization carries macro-level problems, too. When the mental health and primary care organizations do not share the same operational and financial risks, benefits, and systems of doing business, there is very little integration, clinically or otherwise. This means neither party benefits fully from the advantages integrated care offers. Research has taught us that partially integrated care, poorly planned integrated care, lack of shared risk-taking by all parties, and poor leadership buy-in hinder the success of integrated care programs.[4, 5]

In summary, ask yourself and your staff the *who, what, where,* and *why* for launching an integrated behavioral healthcare service. This will make it easier for you to find business cases that not only seem reasonable from a financial perspective, but that will be more easily embraced by your staff and patients. Implementing these programs requires change. This preparatory exercise reveals your paths of least and most resistance, which may draw you toward one model of IBH versus another. In the following chapter, we discuss the specific IBH models. Including a description of these models in your staff survey may help you identify the program that is most likely to succeed in your clinic.

References

1. Marvel MK, Epstein RM, Flowers K, Beckman HB. Soliciting the patient's agenda: have we improved? *JAMA*. 1999;20;281(3):283-287. DOI: 10.1001/jama.281.3.283.
2. Carey M, Jones K, Meadows G, Sanson-Fisher R, D'Este C, Inder K et al. Accuracy of general practitioner unassisted detection of depression. *See comment in PubMed Commons belowAust N Z J Psychiatry*. 2014;48(6):571-578. DOI: 10.1177/0004867413520047.
3. See comment in PubMed Commons belowCraven MA, Bland R. Depression in primary care: current and future challenges. *Can J Psychiatry*. 2013;58(8):442-8. http://search.proquest.com/docview/1429243960/accountid=41151. Accessed January 6, 2015.
4. Institute for Healthcare Improvement. *IHI 90-Day R&D Project Final Summary Report: Integrating Behavioral Health and Primary Care*. Cambridge, MA: Institute for Healthcare Improvement; March 2014. Available at www.ihi.org.
5. Scharf DM, Eberhart NK, Hackbarth NS, Horvitz-Lennon M, Beckman R., Han B et al. *Evaluation of the SAMHSA Primary and Behavioral Health Care Integration (PBHCI) Grant Program: Final Report (Task 13)*. 2014; Santa Monica, CA: RAND Corporation. http://www.rand.org/pubs/research_reports/RR546.html. Accessed April 24, 2015.

CHAPTER 4

A Menu of Integrated Behavioral Health Options

BOTTOM LINE, UP FRONT

- Choosing a model of integrated behavioral healthcare (IBH) is perhaps the MOST important step, but understanding a little about these in advance will help you conduct the prerequisite business development steps and begin key discussions with your staff.

- Integrated behavioral health is a rapidly emerging and evolving field, so there may be an inherent level of risk to your initiative no matter how tightly you develop your business plan.

- Integrating behavioral health into primary care brings two very different cultures together under one mission. Many complexities accompany this transition. If you plan accordingly, you will be able to mitigate risks associated with these cultural discrepancies.

- Using a well-established model allows you to start with a base of clinical, administrative, and operational standards that have scientific support. If executed with fidelity, you are more likely to get program outcomes similar to other systems; be able to predict gains, losses and risks; and have a standardized, replicable, and scalable program.

- DO NOT ONLY scour the primary literature and books about integrated mental health models in order to launch your program. The launch will fail, or will take a wasteful amount of time, resources, and money to make it successful. Many large and small healthcare entities have made this mistake. Read on to understand what to do instead.

One common mistake organizations make as they embark on integration is to simply read a book or a few articles in a journal about how integration works—including all its features—and believe that these materials alone will adequately equip the organization to forge a successful integrated primary care program. We have never seen this happen in our collective experience and a recent review of the 56 federally funded grant programs for integrated care drew similar conclusions.[1]

Integrated behavioral health programs require a fundamentally different approach to the delivery of services to people with mental health and health behaviors. These changes include different coding and billing practices, different clinical skill sets, and medical record documentation, as well as different team-based approaches to managing patient healthcare. Many of these details are discussed in Section II of this book.

There is also a gap in the mental health field—in training and experience in the philosophy underlying integrated care, population health concepts, the medical home model, and the Triple Aim, which lie at the heart of our reasons for integrating. This is particularly true for anyone who completed graduate school before the millennium. Notwithstanding this, integrated care concepts are a fairly new paradigm for many seasoned mental healthcare professionals. Despite 30 years of research on these topics, many behavioral health professionals are just learning about them. Consequently, most mental health providers available for hire will need explicit re-specialization training—some more than others. We help you address these hiring and training needs in Chapters 9 and 10. Read on.

Choosing a model of integrated mental health is important. Sure, various studies have tested specific services, models, or components of models. But to make this ship sail, you will need maps, instructional guides, and other tools to integrate all of these programmatic elements in an efficient way. No one wants to pioneer a program that is implemented in an ineffective way. Consider focusing more on how the models function (i.e., what the professional actually *does* with and for the patient and the healthcare team) and less on how they are branded or what they are named.

While there is nothing inherently wrong with simply hiring a behavioral health provider and then following the process described in Chapter 11 for transforming your practice into an integrated one, we believe it's important to give you specific and calibrated tools. These tools come in the form of formal models that have been discussed in the research conceptually, and in some cases, studied empirically. We believe your pace of integrating and likelihood of developing a successful IBH service rests in your ability to implement well-defined models of integration. This also helps you understand the risks and benefits of these models in advance versus having to clumsily learn them along the way.

Although there has been some discussion in the field about what constitutes a unique model and who decides that one model is unique from another, we have boiled it down to the models that operate uniquely and in clearly defined ways. We have selected models with the most research and/or with clear, uniform training standards. Adopting such a model will increase your likelihood of finding the right behavioral health providers (BHPs) for the program you launch.

SERVICE DELIVERY MODELS

There are five formal models you might consider launching.

1. **The Primary Care Behavioral Health Model (PCBH)**—a biopsychosocial approach to population-based clinical healthcare that is simultaneously co-located, collaborative, and integrated within primary care. The goal of PCBH is to improve and promote overall health and mental health (may include substance abuse) within the primary care population. The hallmark of this model is that the BHP serves as a consultant to the PCPs and help patients self-manage their symptoms. This does not provide a level of services equal to outpatient mental health (e.g., psychotherapy), and as such, is not a substitute for those services if they are clinically warranted. The BHP's schedule and practice style mirrors the PCPs' where each appointment is 15 to 30 minutes and up to 16 patients may be seen daily by a BHP. These BHPs also may provide curbside consults, educational classes for patients, or shared medical appointments. Critically, the BHP's recommendations are intended to initiate, enhance, or assist with the PCPs' and patients treatment plans and healthcare goals.

2. **Co-located Specialty Mental Health**—really means the BHP happens to work at the same site as your PCPs, which could be somewhere in the same building, floor, or even wing as the PCPs. This model lacks many elements of integration, including shared treatment planning, documentation, and provider goals; population focus; focus on general health conditions; and published quality metrics. Providers in this model will have the same limited access, small caseloads, and long wait times observed in non-integrated specialty mental health clinics. Finally, it places the burden of collaboration on BHPs who may not have adequate training, skills, and buy-in to accomplish this. Yet, this remains an easy way to begin integration, and many of the tools developed by the Substance Abuse and Mental Health Services Administration (SAMHSA) are geared toward this model.

3. **Medical Family Therapy (MedFT)**—uniquely incorporates a stronger emphasis on patients' individual and social relational context in reference to their health and mental health. Like PCBH, it is also co-located, collaborative, and integrated within primary care. MedFT typically refers to marriage and family therapists who have received additional training in adapting their clinical skills to integrated behavioral health settings. They apply biopsychosocial systems theory to conducting psychotherapy with patients and their families who experience general health or mental health problems, including illness,

trauma, or disability. These professionals may also provide more abbreviated care when time does not permit the specialty level of care it embodies. When time for specialty-based care is not available, these BHPs deliver a brief service more like the PCBH, with the additions of the social relational perspective mentioned above.

4. **Collaborative Care Model (also called a Care Management, Staff Advisor or Care Facilitation Models)**—targets specific diseases for which patients are being prescribed psychotropic medication in order to drive down disease prevalence, contain cost, increase treatment effectiveness and adherence, and access psychiatry consultation services. These services are usually conducted telephonically, making them fairly easy to integrate, since they don't require exam room space. Psychiatry services in primary care may be most helpful if delivered in the context of this model. These are billable. Note that for simplicity, we will use the term Care Management Model to differentiate this model from the others and to avoid confusing this with care which happens to be collaborative or managed. Most of the primary literature refers to this as the Collaborative Care Model.

5. **Bidirectional/Reverse Integration**—often supported by mental health and substance abuse administrations within states in an attempt to meet quality improvement through integrated care for specific seriously and persistently mentally ill or other identified populations. This model typically is limited in scope, breadth, and depth of integration. Its hallmark is hiring a PCP to work inside a specialty mental health clinic. There is benefit to this model, particularly for patients having severe mental illness, who tend to die younger and often do not receive primary care services routinely.

Table 4.1 (see pages 38 and 39) compares and contrasts these models. We have done our best to whittle this chart down to the most important factors that might interest you in selecting one or more models for implementation. We also acknowledge that there are books written that include some instruction on most of these models and we encourage you to peruse these if it helps you make a decision about which model is best for you.

All of these models can use standard (and free) clinical outcome instruments to gauge the clinical progress of patients. These measures are short and appropriate for primary care. This will bear more relevance for you when you read Section II and explore your preferences for monitoring the outcomes of your program. Add a mental bookmark about this issue, so you can select outcome instruments that meet your patient care and business needs.

FINAL THOUGHTS

While it is probably easiest to envision providing a specialty level of mental healthcare within your primary care clinic (co-located specialty mental health), this model carries most of the same limitations of the mental health system itself (See Chapter 1): a limited population focus (a small subset of the entire population of patients who can benefit); limited access (i.e., 5–8 patients/day); variable quality; and inability to address the majority of patients' needs. While some tout this as a "good start," this approach is exceedingly difficult to introduce due to the lack of shared mission and culture between specialty mental healthcare and primary care.

Moreover, phasing out a co-located specialty mental health program and transitioning to a more fully integrated model also presents significant problems. Changing these business rules and clinical services confuses patients and primary care staff, while changing the function or purpose of the integrated BHP from specialty level (i.e., hour-long, weekly, uninterruptable, highly intensive appointments) to a primary level (i.e., brief, as-indicated, flexible, educational and self-care driven). Many BHPs will not welcome this new role, particularly if they were hired under the former set of rules and treatment intensity.

It is possible to launch co-located specialty mental health programs and even transition them to other integrated models. But be prepared for unavoidable challenges, such as firing incumbent BHPs and re-training or hiring new ones, re-training staff, re-educating patients, and re-working your business plan. Also know that if this is your most viable path to integration, there are several tools published by SAHMSA to assist you and a recent RAND report,[1] which shares some lessons learned from grant-funded programs who have implemented co-located specialty mental health models.

While some systems have tried to have their co-located mental health provider conduct both specialty and primary levels of care, having one single provider deliver care following both models can be very challenging. Standards of care and scopes of practice may become mixed and confused, leading to potential legal liabilities, and patient and provider dissatisfaction. We have only seen this work in exceptional circumstances.

In summary, co-located specialty mental health is certainly one plausible option for integration, but it may not deliver the results you seek from integration, and there are some clear drawbacks. If another model seems to be a reasonable alternative after developing your business plan, consider implementing that alternative.

Finally, we considered adding health coaching to the list of service-delivery models. Health coaching components may include increasing patient motivation (i.e., motivational interviewing and stages of change), educating patients, helping patients set goals for treatment, and increasing accountability and follow-up on patients' goals and the treatment plans.[4-12] Peer support and peer mentoring[6] are two other types of health coaching that provide patients with social support and accountability in pursuit of improving treatment adherence and self-management.

TABLE 4.1. Comparing Five Formal Service Delivery Models of Integrated Behavioral Health

Service Delivery Model	Practice Level	Third-Party Payment Ease	Training Needed	Services Included and Problems Treated
PCBH	Provider	Fairly easy; state-by-state differences for treating general health conditions	Some training needed; very little training needed if hiring a clinical health psychologist or someone whose degree is specialized in primary care integration	Mental health, some substance abuse, and any general health condition that behavioral medicine helps; services include education and self-management skills with patient
Co-located specialty mental health	Provider	Easy. Requires ensuring provider is on all panels needed for reimbursement	None beyond graduate level of education; familiarity with primary care culture needed	Mostly mental health and some substance abuse; services involve psychotherapy if hiring a non-psychiatric prescriber; may include medication management (i.e., "shared care" in Canada) if hiring a psychiatrist or psychiatric nurse practitioner
MedFT	Provider	Fairly easy; state-by-state differences for treating general health conditions; family therapy is not reimbursed by most third-party payers	Some training needed	Family psychotherapy preferred; family issues as they relate to general or mental health and some substance abuse issues; when time does not permit, these BHPs may also do brief work (i.e., help patients self-manage symptoms)
Care Management	Non-provider	More difficult; varies by state; nurse time may be paid by third party, but psychiatric prescriber's services are not; "shared care" delivered by psychiatrists are widely paid by third parties	A little training is needed; more training needed if service will include helping patients self-manage symptoms	Telephonic medication management monitoring and treatment adherence by nurse; any mental health problem for which medications are the first-line treatment; part-time psychiatric prescriber serving a consultation and liaison function
Reverse/Bidirectional Integration	PCP Provider	Easy when there are state and federal grants available	BHP training is needed on physical health conditions; PCP training on mental health conditions is needed; shared language, communication, and team-based care training	Primary care services delivered in a behavioral health setting (e.g., community mental health center; federally qualified behavioral health home)

Research Support	Caseload Size	Role of BHP and PCP	Comments
Some empirical, theoretical and conceptual research; observational studies	Published guidelines advise up to 16 patients per day and population containing at least 3K to 10K patients	BHP does not "own" the patients; care is adjunct to PCPs' treatment plans; all visits last 15 to 30 minutes and are solution-focused	A versatile model; training is available in university and non-university settings; does not provide specialty level of mental healthcare—only the primary level (i.e., helps patients self-manage their symptoms); very collaborative with PCPs
None for psychotherapy delivered in this capacity; "shared care" has some empirical, theoretical, and conceptual research	No published guidelines available; no more than 8 patients usually seen in an 8-hour day	BHP "owns" his/her patients and may work independently of PCP; PCP may have more oversight in "shared care" models; visits last 30 to 60 minutes	Probably the easiest to start; least extent of integration; may increase patients attending first appointment but creates a bottleneck for access; little teamwork between PCP and BHP required; most BHPs practicing this model lack skills needed to work in an integrated way
Some theoretical and conceptual research	No published guidelines available; likely between 8 and 16 patients per day	BHP may "own" patients but will operate very collaboratively with PCPs; visits last 15-60 minutes and may involve family members—depending on patient need and time available	A versatile specialty—not a separate model in and of itself as it delivers specialty and primary levels of care; training is available only within university degree programs
Empirical, theoretical and conceptual research; experimental studies (high-quality, randomized controlled trials)	No published guidelines, but recommended for patient population over 3K and common caseloads have been 80 patients; if optimized and streamlined 150 to 300 may be possible	BHP does not "own" the patients, care is directed by PCPs and managed by nurses	Narrow model of integration; organized around a specific disease; psychiatric prescribing advisor can be located outside the clinic when performing consultation and liaison role
Some theoretical and conceptual research	No published guidelines, but one PCP is usually integrated to implement basic primary care services		Only helpful if your population involves severe mentally ill patients AND you are responsible for providing their mental healthcare

Unfortunately, there is no standard definition, training, or certification for health coaching to help practice leaders and managers or integrated program directors predict and control quality. Consequently, we concur with the literature that health coaching is not so much a distinct model of behavioral health integration as it is an explicit function or task that a professional, paraprofessional, or peer accomplishes when working with patients.[4,5] Some national experts recommend a "health coaching role" as an important skillset one can use for better care with high-utilizing chronically ill patients.[9,13] As such, instead of hiring personnel who only provide health coaching, some organizations have trained their medical assistants, licensed professional nurses, registered nurses, and PCPs to provide health coaching as a routine method for implementing all treatment plans.[4,5,14] A properly trained BHP will already have training in health coaching. We concur with these practices and encourage this approach if health coaching is desired.

References

1. Scharf DM, Eberhart NK, Hackbarth NS, Horvitz-Lennon M, et al. *Evaluation of the SAMHSA Primary And Behavioral Health Care Integration (PBHCI) Grant Program: Final Report (Task 13)*. Santa Monica, CA: RAND Corporation; 2014. http://www.rand.org/pubs/research_reports/RR546.html. Accessed April 24, 2015.
2. Ware JE, Kosinski M, Keller SD. A 12-item short-form health survey: construction of scales and preliminary tests of reliability and validity. *Med Care*. 1996;34(3):220-233. http://journals.lww.com/lww-medicalcare/Abstract/1996/03000/A_12_Item_Short_Form_Health_Survey__Construction.3.aspx. Accessed July 6, 2015.
3. Krebs EE, Lorenz KA, Blair MJ, et al. Development and initial validation of the PEG, a three-item scale assessing pain intensity and interference. *J Gen Intern Med*. 2009;24(6):733-738. http://link.springer.com/article/10.1007/s11606-009-0981-1. Accessed July 6, 2015.
4. Bennett HD, Coleman EA, Parry C, Bodenheimer TA, Chen EH. Health coaching for Patients with chronic illness. *Fam Pract Manag*. 2010;17(5): 24-29. http://www.aafp.org/fpm/2010/0900/p24.html. Accessed January 13, 2015.
5. Bodenheimer T, Laing BY. The teamlet model of primary care. *Ann Fam Med*. 2007;5(5):457-461. DOI: 10.1370/afm.731.
6. Thom DH, Ghorob A, Hessler D, De Vore D, Chen E, Bodenheimer TA. Impact of peer health coaching on glycemic control in low-income patients with diabetes: a randomized controlled trial. *Ann Fam Med*. 2013; 11(2):137-144. DOI: 10.1370/afm.1443.
7. Norris SL, Engelgau MM, Narayan KM. Effectiveness of self-management training in type 2 diabetes: a systematic review of randomized controlled trials. *Diabetes Care*. 2001; 24(3):561-587. DOI: 10.2337/diacare.24.3.561.
8. Linden A, Butterworth SW, Prochaska JO. Motivational interviewing-based health coaching as a chronic care intervention. *J Eval Clin Pract*. 2010;16(1):166-174. DOI: 10.1111/j.1365-2753.2009.01300.x.
9. Olsen JM, Nesbitt BJ. Health coaching to improve healthy lifestyle behaviors: an integrative review. *Am J Health Promot*. 2010;25(1):e1–e12. DOI: 10.4278/ajhp.090313-LIT-101.
10. Lanese BS, Dey A, Srivastava P, Figler R. Introducing the health coach at a primary care practice: impact on quality and cost (Part 1). *Hosp Top*. 2011;89(1):16-22. DOI: 10.1080/00185868.2011.550207.
11. Lanese BS, Dey A, Srivastava P, Figler R. Introducing the health coach at a primary care practice: a pilot study (Part 2). *Hosp Top*. 2011;89(2):37-42 DOI: 10.1080/00185868.2011.572800.

12. Wadden TA, Volger S, Sarwer DB, Vetter ML, Tsai AG, Berkowitz, RI et al. A two-year randomized trial of obesity treatment in primary care practice. *N Engl J Med*. 2011;24;365(21):1969-1979. DOI: 10.1056/NEJMoa1109220.
13. Mautner DB, Pang H, Brenner JC, Shea JA, et al. Generating hypotheses about care needs of high utilizers: lessons from patient interviews. *Popul Health Manag*. 2013;16 Suppl:S26-S33. DOI: 10.1089/pop.2013.0033.
14. National Committee for Quality Assurance (NCQA). *2014 PCMH Standards and Guidelines*. 2014. http://store.ncqa.org/index.php/2014-pcmh-standards-and-guidelines-epub-single-user.html. Accessed December 15, 2014.

SECTION II

Business Development, Policy, and Operations

CHAPTER 5
Policy

> **BOTTOM LINE, UP FRONT**
>
> - Having a detailed policy on integrated behavioral health (IBH) provides a framework for standard operating procedures the entire organization uses for the overarching concepts and specific details of all necessary program components.
>
> - Effective initiation and maintenance of IBH services are at risk for failure if there is not an individual or committee responsible for oversight of effective policy implementation.
>
> - Development of a clinical practice manual ensures the IBH service has a distinct set of operationally defined/benchmark practices that provide a road map of integrated care and clinical and administrative behavior.
>
> - No matter how good an IBH idea might be, without support from leadership and a subsequent sense of ownership and participation from all members of the team, it has a good chance of failing.

Oh joy, our favorite thing in healthcare: *policy*. While many people may have a negative response when they hear the word *policy*, in this context, policy (as you define it) is your friend. Having a detailed policy for IBH in your practice/system is the foundation upon which a successful start-up program is based. It is the black and white communication source document and set of rules that anyone in the organization can reference for overarching as well as specific details on all the necessary components of your program.[1,2]

Furthermore, research shows that implementation demands practice and policy changes at various levels (e.g., service delivery, information exchange, healthcare workforce, financing of care, quality oversight), and that multidimensional efforts to improve IBH are more likely to achieve positive results.[3,4] Assigning responsibility and accountability to members of the delivery system providing the integrated behavioral healthcare can improve the overall success of the program.[1]

THE IMPORTANCE OF A DETAILED PLAN

While policy certainly should be matched to the goals of your IBH services, there are some standard components that everyone should consider including. Answers to the following questions can help make the first draft of that policy as easy as possible. You put your best foot forward if you use your business case analysis (BCA) and business plan to help answer these questions. The business strategy outlined in the next section also will guide this process, as some of these questions are determined by the answers to preceding questions.

1. Who is responsible for overseeing compliance with policy and ensuring funds, training, system rollout of services, and program evaluation are done according to policy? Effective initiation and maintenance of IBH services are at risk for failure if there is not an individual or committee responsible for oversight of effective policy implementation.
2. What clinical practice service manual(s) (i.e., standard operating procedures [SOPs]) need to be developed and what content needs to be included (e.g., forms, clinical tools, administrative tools)?
3. What staffing ratio will you maintain (e.g., 1 BHP per every 7500 enrollees or 1 nurse care manager for every 10,000 enrollees)?
4. What model(s) of service delivery are going to be used (See Chapter 4)? Describe the main components of those models in the policy.
5. What kind of credential will you require for your BHP or medical family therapist (e.g., psychologist, social worker, licensed marriage and family therapist, licensed professional counselor); health coach (e.g., college graduate, peer); complementary and alternative medicine (CAMS) provider (e.g., college degree plus certification in mindfulness, yoga); or care manager/facilitator (e.g., registered or licensed professional nurse, medical technician)?
6. What type of training/skills do behavioral health personnel need to have in order to work effectively in your system? (See Chapter 10 for details/recommendations for training.)
7. What type of enrollees will they be working with (e.g., adult, child, everyone, only those with a particular diagnosis)?
8. What type of screening/assessment will be done?
9. What services will not be included in IBH?

For an example of this type of policy, see the Military Health System (MHS) Web site: www.dtic.mil/whs/directives/corres/pdf/649015p.pdf. This MHS policy covers services for 3.3 million individuals in more than 300 adult medical home primary care clinics. We believe their material can easily be adapted to your specific needs.

The Partners in Health: Mental Health, Primary Care and Substance Use Interagency Collaboration Tool Kit, 2nd ed. (2013), from SAMHSA, is another source that can be helpful in drafting policy documents—especially the

Interagency Agreements section. The tool kit can be found at: www.ibhp.org/uploads/file/IBHPIinteragency%20Collaboration%20Tool%20Kit%202013%20.pdf

SOPS: A CLINICAL PRACTICE MANUAL

Standard operating procedures (SOPs) build from the policy documents. They provide the specifics of *how* the IBH program will do *what* the policy says must be done. Existing medical home concepts can be incorporated easily into IBH SOPs. Your branding and marketing strategy may be best if you integrate IBH SOPs into one document with other medical home SOPs.

> *Include in your manual, information all stakeholders can use, so everyone can understand their roles in reference to the other team members and facets of the program.*

A clinical practice manual is another important structural document for IBH service delivery. It includes a distinct set of operationally defined/benchmark practices that provide a road map of IBH clinical and administrative behavior. Include in your manual, information all stakeholders can use, so everyone can understand their roles in reference to the other team members and facets of the program. We realize that the size and complexity of your organization, funding, and program goals will determine which stakeholders are included in this document. To be *most* comprehensive, a practice manual should include the following:

I. **Guidelines, Goals, and Objectives**
   A. The Role of Behavioral Health in Integrated Primary Care
   B. Integrated Behavioral Health Model (the one(s) you choose to launch)
   C. Key Principles of Integrated Care
   D. Program Goals and Evaluation Processes (may include metrics you devise when reading Chapter 8)

II. **Roles and Responsibilities of the Integrated Care Team**
   A. Integrated Care Team Member: Primary Care Provider
   B. Integrated Care Team Member: Medical Assistant
   C. Integrated Care Team Member: Alternative and Complementary Medicine Provider
   D. Integrated Care Team Member: Behavioral Health Consultant or Medical Family Therapist
   E. Integrated Care Team Member: Care Facilitator
   F. Integrated Care Team Member: Registered Nurse

G. Integrated Care Team Member: Psychiatric Consultant
H. Integrated Care Team Member: Licensed Professional Nurse
I. Integrated Care Leadership: Integrated Care Program Lead
J. Integrated Care Leadership: Clinic Site Director
K. Integrated Care Leadership: Integrated Care Clinical Supervisor
L. Integrated Care Resources: Integrated Care Advisor
M. Integrated Care Resources: Integrated Care Committee
N. Integrated Care Recipient: Patients and Their "Bill of Rights"

III. **Training Program (or Requirements) Overview**
   A. Didactic Training
   B. Core Competency Training
   C. Self-Directed Learning
   D. Sustainment Training and Ongoing Learning

IV. **Clinical Activities**
   A. Clinical Services of Integrated Care Team
      1. Brief Interventions
      2. Clinical Pathway Programs
      3. Step-up/Step-down Pathway Programs
      4. Excluded Services
   B. Practice Support Tools
      1. Primary Care Provider/Other Team Member Referral Scripts
      2. Primary Care Provider/Other Team Member Referral Form
      3. Clinical Guides for the Behavioral Health Professional
      4. Clinical Guides for the (all other team members)
   C. Outcome Assessment Tools and Screeners
      1. Recommended Routine Outcome Tools (See Chapter 8 for ideas)
      2. Recommended Routine Screening Tools for all Medical Home Patients
      3. Recommended "As-Indicated" Screening Tools
   D. Clinical Policies and Procedures
      1. Patient Access to the Behavioral Health Professional
      2. Patient Involvement in the Integrated Care Committee
      3. Informed Consent
      4. Clinical Assessment Standards
   E. Quality Assurance of Charting and Documentation
   F. Providing Feedback to the Primary Care Provider
   G. Medication Consultations with Primary Care Providers and Patients
   H. Psychiatric Consultations with Primary Care Providers and Patients
   I. Telemedicine

V. Administrative Procedures
  A. Appointment Templates (per Integrated Care Team member, as you may launch two different models or have a separate role for each BHP)
  B. Coding
  C. Revenue/Billing
  D. Performance Measures /Quality Metrics
  E. Staffing Guidelines
  F. Productivity Standards
  G. Core Competency Skills (for each Integrated Care Team member)

An easily modifiable sample practice manual that includes these topic areas and may be adapted for PCBH and MedFT models of IBH can be found at www.pcpci.org/pcbh-implementation-kit-library.

For those interested in SOPs/clinical practice manuals/guidance for a Care Management Model of serviced delivery for depression go to http://impact-uw.org/tools.

LEADERSHIP APPROVAL AND FUNCTIONAL SUPPORT

What? You mean everyone doesn't think this is a good idea? No matter how good an IBH idea might be, if all players on the team (e.g., medical technician, nurses, physicians, program administrators, financial and other executive personnel) are not engaged and if they don't feel a sense of ownership, it has a good chance of failing. Practical experience from multiple systems[1,2] have consistently shown that the following are important for success:

1. Include finance, personnel, and management individuals in the program development process. The program must be fundable (See Chapters 3, 6, 7; Appendices 6B-6D; Tables 6.2, 6.3; and Section III), and various levels of management must fully support the program for there to be a chance of success. See Table 5.1 for a review of specific key stakeholders and *how* they may support integrated care.
2. Identify and assign a behavioral health and a medical home champion who are respected and can represent the views of the professionals who work in their clinics. These individuals also should be able to speak the language of finance, personnel, and management to help facilitate a common approach moving forward. Having a strong healthcare advocate who informs others with real-world stories, scientific data, and potential return on investment will facilitate movement of the clinical and operational worlds in the same direction.
3. Ensure that the rationale for establishing integrated care is clear, evidence-based, or evidence-informed (see IBH models [Chapter 4]); considers your goals (Chapter 3); is based on solid business case analyses (Chapter 6);, and explicitly defines the operational and financial barriers your system faces.

TABLE 5.1. Integrated Care Development Key Stakeholders for Support

Professional Title	Role in Supporting Integrated Care Development
Chief Executive Officer (CEO)	Support of program at highest level. Recognition of need to change culture of system to integrated care; larger vision development. Representative of integrated care at larger systems level and within legislation and networking.
Chief Operations Officer (COO)	Support for the daily operations and overall development of integrated care within the organization.
Chief Financial Officer (CFO)	Support for fiscal development. Identification of pro formas, financial cost/benefit ratios, and financial planning to support integrated care development throughout system. Support for direct and indirect revenues and grant development.
Executive Team / Board of Directors	Support for overall implementation and vision. Consideration of behavioral health representation at executive team level.
Quality Improvement	Support for clinical quality metrics and implementation of integrated care through medical home, HEDIS, and/or specific clinical quality metrics.
Medical Director Director of Nursing Director of Behavioral Health/Mental Health/Substance Abuse services	Support for integrated care at a practice-based level. Support for behavioral assessment and treatment of medical conditions, population health management, referral management, and use of behavioral health support as a member of the care team. Development of workflows for care management with behavioral health providers.
Billing Department	Support for integrated care assessment and treatment coding, dual and same-day visits, and additional types of direct revenue.
Information Technology Lead/Electronic Medical Records Lead	Support for shared communication and documentation within medical records. Support for data elements/data pulls for continuous quality improvement (CQI), model fidelity management, and quality assurance.
Site Provider Champions	Support for integrated care at a practice-based level. Support within staff meetings, referral management, and identification/recognition of behavioral health as primary care team member. Support to provide education and encouragement as champions of the model.
Other Site-Specific Support	Support for integrated care at a practice-based level. Administrative and clinical support to practice and operate integrated care.
Patient Advisory Boards / Community	Support from patients and community related to how they will utilize behavioral health within primary care and their plan to request services as an expectation of quality standard care.
Community and State-Level Stakeholders	Support for implementing integrated care from a Triple Aim and population health perspective.

4. Carefully determine when to present proposals to those who make the final decisions. Proceed only when there is a clear rationale/argument to be made and the decision-makers' questions can be answered in thoughtful and informative ways.
5. For additional ideas about securing buy-in from leadership, or convincing yourself that these models are beneficial (since you may be one of the leaders), see the section entitled "Why Some Administrators Don't Want Mental Health Patients" in Chapter 6.

References

1. Scharf DM, Eberhart NK, Hackbarth NS, Horvitz-Lennon M, Beckman R., Han B et al. *Evaluation of the SAMHSA Primary and Behavioral Health Care Integration (PBHCI) Grant Program: Final Report (Task 13)*. Santa Monica, CA: RAND Corporation; 2014. http://www.rand.org/pubs/research_reports/RR546.html. Accessed April 24, 2015.
2. Hunter CL, Goodie JL. Behavioral health in the Department of Defense Patient-Centered Medical Home: history, finance, policy, work force development, and evaluation. *Transl Behav Med*. 2012;2(3): 355-363. DOI: 10.1037/a0021761.
3. Horvitz-Lennon M, Kilbourne AM, Pincus HA. From silos to bridges: meeting the general health care needs of adults with severe mental illnesses. *Health Aff*. 2006;25(3):659-669. DOI: 10.1377/hlthaff.25.3.659.
4. Institute of Medicine (US). Committee on Crossing the Quality Chasm: Adaptation to Mental Health and Addictive Disorders. *Improving the quality of health care for mental and substance-use conditions*. Washington, DC: National Academy Press; 2006.

CHAPTER 6
Business Development

BOTTOM LINE, UP FRONT

- The more access you have to data about your patients, practice, financial flow, and payers, the more well-equipped you will be to develop a strong business plan.
- Because there is such diversity in healthcare organization types and revenue sources, your business plan will be determined by the type of organization you are: large, self-contained system (e.g., state or federal government, healthcare management organization); Accountable Care Organization (ACO); Federally Qualified Health Center (FQHC); hospital-based practice; or small private practice.
- Figure 6.1 can help you with your overarching business strategy; it is designed to prevent you from making costly mistakes as you launch.
- Carefully review activities, demands, and patients' needs in your current practice.
- Make an effort to identify reimbursement approaches, which are variable and specific to your type of organization, state, and local (e.g., county) laws and payers' policies.
- Electronic health records and electronic medical records are the cornerstone for improved internal management of the patient between his or her medical home team and the rest of the practice.
- Viable business cases and a well-thought-out business plan for integrated behavioral health care (IBH) are ways to a secure future based on quality of care and fiscal sustainability.
- Consider diversifying your revenue streams in order to sustain your program as it matures and the current healthcare landscape continues to shift.

Much of the content in this chapter addresses business strategy and development, viable payment models, service structure and delivery, and data management. The latter topic drives all the former ones. Historically, the business of paying for behavioral health services has been one of the toughest challenges in launching IBH because policies and laws continually change. Therefore, we have devised several tools that will help you sustain operations even as this landscape shifts, regardless of the size or type of your organization. Wherever a business development concept or tool carries particular relevance for one organization type versus another, we have specified that for your convenience.

Some of your skeptical colleagues have avoided establishing formal business plans or clinical programs for addressing primary care patients' mental health needs.

What we have heard in the field:

"As an administrator I don't want to have to deal with patients who need mental health services. And here is why . . .
- There are various issues with payment; insurances don't cover all services.
- We have to try to collect what we can. Even with a discount, collection of patient money is a problem.
- They take too much time when seeing our providers, making it more difficult for our providers to maintain their schedules.
- They are substance abusers and bring their bad habits and unsavory appearances into our reception area.
- They are doctor shoppers and seek medication from anyone they can find.
- Our cost benefit analysis of treating them due to time and poor reimbursement do not make it worthwhile.
- There is a mental health center down the street—we provide care for physical health.
- There are churches and other organizations that can take care of them.
- I don't have enough time in my day to think about or worry about these types of patient issues."

We realize the mindset of some administrators is a function of their experiences in a particular system, and they might not be willing to disclose these perspectives publically—all of which is understandable. But these are not good reasons to avoid integrating behavioral healthcare in your medical home. If these sentiments do not reflect your concerns and perspective, skip to the section below. However, if any of them are an obstacle to IBH service development, read Appendix 6A. There, you will find a list of solutions to help you work through the obstacles to IBH. These solutions may help you better understand some of the operational

Chapter 6—Business Development

aspects of an IBH program launch. After reading Appendix 6A, come back here and continue reading.

BUSINESS DEVELOPMENT STRATEGY

One easy way for us to outline a viable business development strategy is illustrated in the flowchart (Figure 6.1), which includes five important steps. Regardless how long ago you launched your IBH service or how long it will be until you launch it, you may consider making significant changes at any step in this process (e.g., hiring different clinicians, pursuing FQHC status). For most organizations, Step One is fairly fixed: the type of healthcare organization you are.

The steps of the flowchart have been arranged so that each step is dependent on the steps preceding it. Each step in the progression generally offers more choices for the organization than the step before. For example, you may not be able to change the type of healthcare institution you are (Step One), but you may

**BUILDING A SUSTAINABLE INTEGRATED BEHAVIORAL HEALTH PROGRAM:
5 START-UP STEPS FOR SUCCESSFUL PLANNING**

HEALTH CARE INSTITUTION SITE LICENSURE
(What type of heathcare institution are you? (e.g., Hospital, Outpatient Treatment Center, Home Health Agency, Behavioral Health, General, Hospice, etc.)

This helps identify state office of administrative counsel rule making regarding your facility.

Action: Review your state laws: Are you legally able to offer integrated care services? Do you need to complete a state application if you are preparing to offer CMS services?

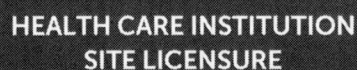

SITE TYPE
(How is your site classified? (e.g., ACO, FQHC, RHC, hospital, etc.)

This helps identify the way you can receive reimbursement, health savings, and outcome measurements. Fiscal direct pro forma as well as return on investment and cost savings are primarily dependent on site type.

Action: What type of healthcare entity are you? Are there rules, regulations, and support for your specific entity for integration? Do you have or wish to develop PCMH? Do you report specific behavioral metrics already related to chronic health conditions and behavioral health (HEDIS, NCQA, Joint Commission, PQRS, Uniform Data System [UDS])?

FIGURE 6.1. (continued on next page)

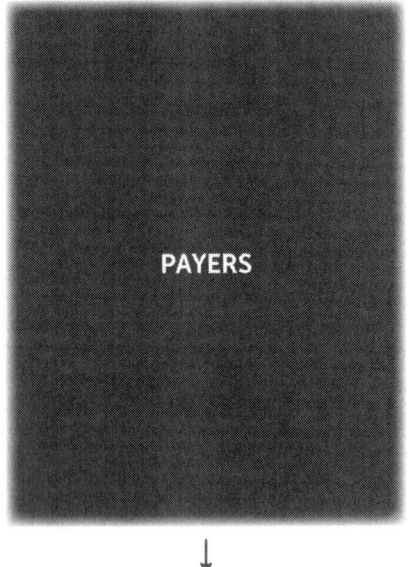

This helps identify reimbursement (service types, program types), health savings, and outcome measurements needed for sustainability.

In addition, payers identify the licensure, regulations, and documentation requirements of providers, services, and programs. Payers also identify the services they need.

Action: Review state and federal regulations related to providing integrated care. What billing options do you have and how do those dictate your program creation (services, providers, billing, documentation, etc.)? Review the private payer's regulations and rules related to providing integrated care. Review your payers (patients') needs for integrated care (reports on diagnoses, chronic medical conditions, screening needs, specialty needs, and interest in behavioral care).

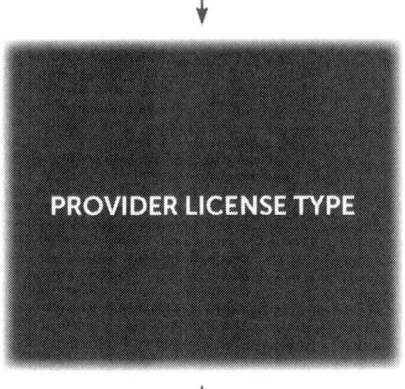

Provider license types identify the areas of specialty, education, training, and professional practice. In addition, licenses are related to reimbursement.

Action: Now that you know what license types are legally able to provide reimbursable care in your center and from whom, create a list of training, documentation, and metrics for integrated care. In addition, identify the business cost of these professionals and the pro forma related to billing and/or cost savings for monitoring.

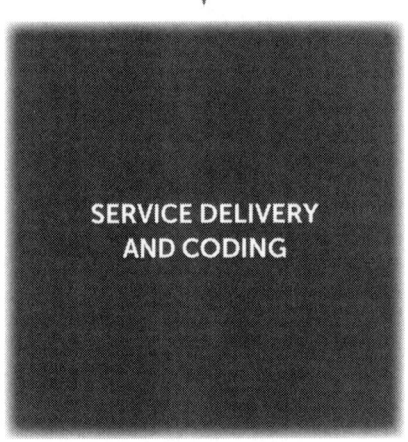

It is essential to identify the service delivery and the available coding per institution, site, payer, and license.

Action: Now that you know the above information, identify the specific CPT codes you can use for the services and providers you plan to incorporate. Create auditing tools to ensure the interventions and documentation meet expectations (continuity and quality care). Also, be aware of your state regulations and interpretations of confidentiality as they apply to mental health and substance abuse services, programs, and interventions. Ensure you are strategic in your verbiage and service delivery.

FIGURE 6.1. (from previous page)

be able to find additional payers (Step Three), and you will definitely be able to choose the services you deliver (Step Five). However, you cannot feasibly start at the last step—choosing what you want to code and bill for—and then decide who your payers will be.

Consider spending a few minutes thinking through these five steps. Using this model as your overarching business strategy may be helpful even as you dig into the details of things like coding and data management. Maintain awareness of where you are in this progression and refer back to this flowchart periodically.

MAKING THE BUSINESS CASE

A 2014 report[1] made economic savings calculations for integrated care. These are depicted in Table 6.1. Another report provides real-world examples of cost savings, (see Table 7.3). These examples of cost savings for treating mental health conditions that co-occur with general health conditions may appeal most to the ACOs and larger, self-contained healthcare organizations, as well as those systems that are interested in reverse integration. In short, the cost savings are out there for the taking. But forging a path to realize these savings remains challenging to many who are interested in launching IBH programs.

TABLE 6.1. Economic Impact of Integrated Medical-Behavioral Healthcare (Melek, Norris, & Paulus, 2014)

Payer	Annual Estimated Cost Savings
Commercial	$15–$31.6 billion
Medicare	$3.3–$6.7 billion
Medicaid	$7.1–9.9 billion
Total	**$26.3–$48.3 billion**

Whether you are a large, self-contained healthcare organization, ACO, or FQHC, developing the business case for IBH requires that you ask a few more questions. Follow Table 6.2 to work through your business case analysis. You will need to consult your organization's records to mine much of this information, and if you do not have extensive or easily accessible records, consider reading this whole chapter, including the sections on Reporting, Management of Data, and Documentation, before developing your business case analysis (BCA).

In Appendix 6B we list several formulas for BCAs. We chose the screening and prevention billing codes for this example because all of the IBH models will be able to do this, making this analysis doable for you no matter which model you implement. Additionally, see Appendix 6C, "Sample Case Study: Hale Health Center," used in the SAMHSA-HRSA Center for Integrated Health Solutions publication, *The Business Case for the Integration of Behavioral Health and Primary Care*[2] which

TABLE 6.2. Developing Your Business Case

Questions	Data Mining
"Is there a patient population in my practice that is not being treated?"	• Diagnoses across the population • Your performance on HEDIS metrics • PQRS
"Is there a patient population in my practice that is being treated in a sub-standard manner?"	• Health maintenance completion rates* • Yearly visit completion corresponding to diagnosis • Diagnosis associated with referred services • Population health (predominant populations treated by diagnosis)* • Quality improvement and clinical performance metrics (e.g., HEDIS, UDS, etc.) • PCMH NCQA metrics
"Is there a patient population in my practice that is being treated in a way that takes time away from other patients due to their comorbid mental health difficulties?"	• CPT coding • Diagnosis coding • Next available appointments • Duplicated vs. unduplicated patients • PQRS • Clinical performance metrics
"Are providers dedicating large amounts of time to complex duplicated patients each week?"	• Duplicated vs. unduplicated patients seen monthly • CPT coding • Diagnosis coding • High-utilizing patients**
"Are patients following through with recommendations for behavioral, mental, or psychiatric assistance?"	• Referral completion logs for behavioral, mental, and psychiatric care referrals • Repeated referrals for the same diagnosis within a given period of time

*These are required to maintain your health and are metrics in healthcare (e.g., flu shot, annual exams, etc.; or population-specific requirements such as diabetes foot exam yearly, mammograms, colonoscopies, etc.)
** Identification of specific patients who visit PCPs $\geq$ 2x/month vs. patients who receive care $\leq$ 1x/month

applies these BCA formulas to a practice so you can put the information in a real-world context. For additional assistance, we recommend going to the following Web site to download an Excel file that has been programed to compute your BCA using the formula in this section: www.integration.samhsa.gov/resource/the-business-case-for-the-integration-of-behavioral-health-and-primary-care

DEVELOPING A BASIC BUSINESS PLAN

Once you've answered the questions in Table 6.2, you will be able to select one or more of these cases or business purposes for implementing IBH. Your BCA results will help you develop vital concepts that you will incorporate into your business plan. If you also are exploring additional sources of financing for developing your IBH program, we list tools for financing in Appendix 6D.

Now, let's move on to the matter of developing your business plan. Although the structure and content of business plans vary and also exceed the scope of this text, we have included some resources in Table 6.3. Irrespective of the model of IBH you launch, all of the questions listed in Table 6.3 are important ones to consider. We have also included possible "answer" sources to make it easier for you to complete. Consider answering the questions listed therein. When combined with your BCAs, the aggregate data should assist you in making the important business decisions around preparing and designing a sustainable IBH product line.

TABLE 6.3. Business Planning Questions You Might Consider

Facet of the Business Plan	Questions to Ask	Sources of Possible Answers
Objectives	• Can we meet a growing need in the community or within our empaneled population? • Can we provide comprehensive care to go beyond our basic approach to patients? • Can we achieve financial benefit? • Can we offer something new that patients are willing to help pay for?	• Key organizational goals • Needs assessment • Identify clinical and organizational value beyond direct revenue • Link to current mission • Triple Aim
Market Analysis and Competitive Analysis	• Is there a need in our community or organization for improved behavioral healthcare services in primary care? • Do we have a need based on our existing patient population or will we need to expand our patient population to fully benefit? • Is there adequate insurance coverage among our patients? • Irrespective of the insurance coverage, are the costs of IBH worth the benefits? • For smaller markets and communities (e.g., rural), what is being done in the other system(s) to meet the mental and behavioral health issues and care needs of our community? • What are the current mental health services offered in the community? • How effective are they at meeting our community's needs? • Can we compete and offer improved care? • What are other local primary care services offering? • What are our health population needs/climate?	• Includes market statistics and trends that will affect your success • Overview of competition and supporters/stakeholders

(Continued on next page)

Facet of the Business Plan	Questions to Ask	Sources of Possible Answers
Product Service / Description	• Do we improve communication and coordination with the existing community providers? • Do we provide space and support services to existing members of the community? • Do we seek an employment arrangement with existing providers? • Do we develop a new program that is unavailable in our community, but achieves better results at a lower expense?	• Comparison of various products and services in detail with respect to community and needs
Operations	• Do we have a champion who will lead the project? • What does our "current state" look like in meeting the needs of our patients and our community? • Do we have space? • Do we have clinical staff and what will it cost? • What support staff will be needed; do we increase current levels? • What changes are required for our information technology structure? • How and what tools will be used to screen patients and to obtain the necessary information? • How much time or support will we offer for current providers by shifting behavioral healthcare to the new program staff members?	• Analysis of strengths, weaknesses, and barriers • Developing management and workflow from top down/bottom up
Financial Analysis	• What will it cost? • What about staffing requirements? • Are we seeking to increase income or offer a service at a worst-case break even? • Will the program contribute to overhead expenses? Do we assign overhead to the program or expect break even on direct outlay of dollars? • What is the payer mix? • What is the employer mix in our community? • Do our existing contracts offer mental health coverage? • Will offering behavioral health services affect our network status? • What payment models do we have in place from fee-for-service to capitation?	• Fiscal costs • Cost offset • Cost savings • Direct reimbursement • Projections • Diversification of funding • Market support

(Continued on next page)

Facet of the Business Plan	Questions to Ask	Sources of Possible Answers
Financial Analysis (continued)	• Will this program be integrated into the contracts and what level/type of reimbursement will be included? • Do we have diversification in our reimbursement systems? • Do we have enough information to develop ROI and cost savings prediction equations?	
Timeframe	• How long will the analysis take? • When can we have a program up and running? • What other projects are happening?	• Strategic plans • Workflows • Organizational plan • Action plan: 1-, 5-, and 10-year
Monitoring	• What key metrics will be reviewed to ensure the program is successful and meeting its objectives? • How will reports be shared with group members? • How will the metrics be generated and supported for data collection and sharing? • What trainings do we need to implement and at what levels and frequency to ensure success? • What supports are needed?	• Link to current regulatory measurements and metrics • Greater services and higher-level regulations for enhanced care (e.g.: PCMH) • Metrics tied to fiscal and objective reporting • Metrics that can be data mined • Relevancy to program • Clinical performance metrics (e.g., PQRS, HEDIS, UDS, registries, etc.) • Medicare Part B claims • Qualified registry • Direct EHR • Certified EHR • Meaningful Use • Wellness, self-management, and goal setting • Collaborative care • Preventive care, screening, health maintenance

DATA REPORTING AND MANAGEMENT

There are a few key points to consider related to reporting and data management in general, but when developing an IBH service, you may want to review and report data weekly and monthly for business operations and revenue flow purposes. First, do you have an electronic medical record (EMR) or electronic health record (EHR)? Often individuals use these terms interchangeably; however, they are defined differently. EMRs were first developed and used within medical offices. These electronic systems are digital versions of paper charts and allow providers to document medical and treatment history, track data easily, and monitor baseline quality of care. The EHR was developed to move beyond basic charting and move practices into improved communication and quality care, while improving patients' abilities to self-manage and be active members of their healthcare.

> **EHRs typically include more thorough data mining capabilities with trending, data analysis/analytics, comparisons, and capabilities to demonstrate health systems meeting the Triple Aim.**

EHR functioning expands practices to reach beyond a provider's medical care to encompass other health professionals, interprofessional healthcare communication, and shared information systems with hospitals, specialists, and laboratories. Further, EHRs are designed to be accessed by patients to improve their education and interaction in their own healthcare, meeting stages of meaningful use. EHRs typically include more thorough data mining capabilities with trending, data analysis/analytics, comparisons, and capabilities to demonstrate health systems meeting the Triple Aim.

Both EMRs and EHRs may be used in practices; however, most organizations are moving toward implementation of EHRs to ensure highest standard of care and federal regulations, including the Patient Protection and Affordable Care Act's (PPACA) Stage 2 Meaningful Use, the Physician Quality Reporting System (PQRS), and the Healthcare Effectiveness Data and Information Set (HEDIS). These electronic record systems are cornerstones for improved internal management of patients between their healthcare team and the practice. If you do not have an EHR, we strongly advise you to invest in one as soon as possible. Without one, your ability to function effectively in the current healthcare climate will become increasingly limited.

An EHR is also critical for IBH. For truly integrated and collaborative care effectiveness, the behavioral health professional must document in the same EHR. However, be aware of certain state-, federal-, and program-specific regulations around sharing of information (limits of confidentiality and release requirements), particularly for substance abuse "programs." For more on this, see the subsection on documentation later in this chapter.

As you build IBH services, you will be collecting and storing more data—data that must be managed effectively. As you know, the EHR data are best used when coupled with data from the practice management system (PMS). Many

EHRs come with interfaced or combined practice management systems for ease. Practice management systems assist with managing, scheduling, billing, and capturing patient data, while complying with the Health Information Technology for Economic and Clinical Health (HITECH) Act. It is best to have a single database—one consolidated system rather than separate EMR and PMS, which would require additional tools for integrating information. Consider these questions:

- Are these one-way or two-way (EMR to PMS, PMS to EMR, or a designed interface in the EHR for bidirectional communication) vehicles?
- How will reports be generated from the data gathered?
- What will the cost be for this process?

We want to highlight that IBH service integration is *not* an additional cost in this area, as your BHP will use the same system you already use. Additionally, it makes mental and behavioral health data readily available for review in the existing system, which adds value and benefit for the patient and primary care team because they have access to complete histories, assessments, and data for improved patient care and collaboration. For further information about selecting a PMS, visit this American Medical Association Web site: www.ama-assn.org/ama/pub/advocacy/topics/administrative-simplification-initiatives/pms-toolkit.page?

If you are in a center that does not have a well-performing PMS or EHR system, you must become resourceful and creative. Many organizations contract for shared PMS and EHR systems, use Web-based services, or outsource administrative processes. No matter how you develop your practice management, it must improve administrative efficiencies, interface with the EHR system, be current with the advances needed to document in healthcare (e.g., "medical home," ICD-10, HIPPA specifications, electronic eligibility, dual scheduling, electronic remittance), and must offer training and ease of use for your practice staff. Further, if your PMS is lacking, carefully consider the extensive benefits of upgrading and ensuring your staff and management are capable with learning healthcare quality management practice and associated IT. This is important not just so you have a solid understanding of your patient population and the details of how your practice operates, but because it also may affect your revenue flow.

For example, consider the PQRS, the quality reporting program that encourages individual eligible professionals (EPs) and group practices to report information on the quality of care to Medicare. As of 2015, the program applies a negative payment adjustment to individual EPs and PQRS group practices that did not satisfactorily report data on quality measures for Medicare Part B Physician Fee Schedule (MPFS)-covered professional services in 2013. Those who report satisfactorily for the 2015 program year avoid the 2017 PQRS negative payment adjustment. There are several PQRS criteria that could be evaluated or considered in the development of internal data and business cases. If you are a Medicare

provider and do not currently monitor these quality data for reporting, you may already be losing money. A few examples relevant to IBH are listed below.
- PQRS #9—Antidepressant Medication Management
- PQRS #106—Adult Major Depression Disorder
- PQRS #173—Unhealthy Alcohol Use
- PQRS #247—Substance Abuse Disorders
- PQRS #134 (NQF 0418): Preventive Care and Screening: Screening for Clinical Depression and Follow-Up Plan (National Quality Strategy Domain: Community/Population Health)

For further information see www.cms.gov/Medicare/Quality-Initiatives-Patient-Assessment-Instruments/PQRS.

> ***If nothing else, a better understanding of your patient population and the services you deliver will help you improve how you run the business and clinical aspects of your practice.***

In many practices, the patient and practice data available for additional business development will be fuzzy at best. In general, we recommend that you approach data analysis and management using the Triple Aim approach to healthcare improvement. (See Chapter 8 for more). However, if your current system is not set up to obtain those data, there may be other sources of data that could help you. Note that data also will help answer your initial or ongoing business case or business development questions. If nothing else, a better understanding of your patient population and the services you deliver will help you improve how you run the business and clinical aspects of your practice. In the next chapter, we include reimbursement considerations for doing this (see the last row of Table 6.3 under "monitoring").

Analyzing your direct current coding and billing statements with specific attention to populations and reimbursable service is a preliminary way to begin developing your business plan. This strategy may be most applicable for medical homes that are smaller, or not FQHCs, ACOs, or grant-funded—those that rely, at least in part, on public and private third-party payers and may have more flexibility to develop a pro forma / business case for integrated care with both direct revenue and cost savings. (See Table 8.3 in Chapter 8 for information on quality metrics you can track for evaluating programs, maximizing billing, and improving your medical home's performance.)

EXPANDING YOUR PROGRAM BEYOND THE BASICS

Once you allocate IBH resources for your patient population, consider the opportunities to leverage these same IBH professionals to increase your market share. If your patients are not visiting the medical home as often (because they are healthier or no longer suffer from a comorbid mental health condition), you can increase the size of your panel. Market, advertise, or do whatever else you can to open enrollment into your clinic. Remember, program development and scaling are essential for long-term vitality; however, they should not be conducted until your IBH program is fully operational and functioning favorably.

The next goal is diversifying your payment structure and patient population. You can start by directly marketing your practice to employers who purchase insurance packages for your payers. These employers may shape their employee healthcare packages with you in mind. Some practices offer primary care and IBH services framed as wellness services (including a registered dietician), while others deliver their IBH services as employee assistance programs (EAPs), providing employees with specialty mental healthcare. Finally, some practices provide specialized behavioral health evaluations that often are associated with or required for certain surgeries and medical tests, such as bariatric surgeries, cochlear implants, spinal cord stimulators, and polysomnography. If your BHP happens to be a clinical health psychologist, very little extra investment will be needed for your practice to develop this aspect of your business, as this area of medical practice is their bailiwick.

References

1. Melek S, Norris D, Paulus J. Economic impact of integrated medical-behavioral healthcare. *Milliman American Psychiatric Association Report*;2014.
2. CSI Solutions LLC. *The Business Case for the Integration of Behavioral Health and Primary Care*. Washington, DC: SAMHSA-HRSA Center for Integrated Health Solutions; 2013. http://www.integration.samhsa.gov/resource/the-business-case-for-the-integration-of-behavioral-health-and-primary-care. Accessed December 18, 2014.

Appendix 6A.
Responses for Administrators Who Don't Want to Serve Patients' Mental Health Needs

Let's take a look at the action points we can assign to each of the concerns we have heard in the field.

- There are issues with payment, insurances don't cover the cost.
  - Mental Health Parity and Addiction Equity Act (MHPAEA) of 2008, and the Patient Protection and Affordable Care Act of 2010, help correct this.
- We have to try to collect what we can, even with a discount collection of patient copays are a problem
  - Update your financial policy within the limits of your site license and all applicable law. Consider adding a statement related to "counseling" patients on payment plans to insure that they understand the importance of meeting their financial obligations.
  - Train the scheduling, reception, and check-out staff on the key aspects of payments for mental health diagnoses. Ideally, when all staff, including billing staff, treat mental health problems the same way they would non-mental health problems, we see the most favorable circumstances. Review the billing tools mentioned in Appendix 7D and Table 7.2 in Chapter 7.
  - Administratively verify the policies of your payers related to mental health diagnoses, including basic coverage and copay amounts. This may also stipulate limits on the number of visits covered. In spite of MHPAEA, as noted, there will be exceptions. See Chapter 7 for a description of these.
  - Ensure all mental health data are managed in the same systems and via the same processes as general health data. There should be few differences as long as local laws permit this.
  - Train your medical billing staff on management of denials, your payers' policies, and the local laws; how to spot denials; and how to address them, including requesting additional information from the payers.
- People with mental health needs take too much time for our providers, messing up the schedule.
  - Leverage your BHP and nurses for screening and follow-up treatment. Remember, the medical home model relies on non-PCP team members.
  - Train the nursing, medical assistants, appointment, and scheduling staff on key terms, phrases, or questions to ask the patient concerning mental health "triggers" in advance so you know these will come up in the patients' visit.

Chapter 6—Business Development

- Use routine screening tools that the front desk, medical assistants, or nurses administer and can be confirmed or addressed when taking vitals in order to discover these problems at the earliest juncture in the patient's visit.
- Implement a clinical pathway so all patients with the same problem are managed in a standardized way.
- Walk the patient in to see your integrated behavioral health professional(s) who will address the behavioral health issues for the PCPs, thereby saving the PCPs time. See workflow suggestions in Chapter 11.
- Many of these patients become the "Oh by the way" type, waiting until after the listed primary reason for visit is complete before addressing their mental health needs. The provider should have the patient walked over to see the BHP.
- They are substance abusers and bring their bad habits and issues into our reception area.
  - Set up a secondary waiting area to shift patients from the main reception area. This can be a private room or an area set aside—perhaps the previous paper chart-filing area! One caveat is to ensure you don't stigmatize these patients and make them feel different. One alternative is to arrange waiting room chairs in rows or other orientations other than lining the perimeter of the room with chairs. This way there are multiple focal points in the room other than the patient who seems to be struggling with a substance abuse issue.
  - Consider special substance use clinics held after hours or at different times of the day. For example, schedule an opioid clinic the last half of the day on the same day each week, when most patients have already left the clinic and when you can devote clinic resources to this specialized population.
  - Shared medical appointments can also be helpful, as these use different space and the patients are immediately moved into the "group room" upon arriving. This provides an extra level of customer service for these particularly sensitive patients, while also leaving the milieu and image of the clinic and waiting room undisturbed. See Chapter 11 for more about shared medical appointments.
- They are doctor shoppers and seek medication from anyone they can find.
  - Set up a tracking mechanism inside the practice to monitor patients on key prescription drugs in the event they move from one doctor to another inside your practice.
  - Devise an agreement with local pharmacies who can help monitor these patient utilization behaviors.
  - Consider the following:

- We (the medical system) provided these patients the medication to which they have become addicted, knowing the risks that these medications pose for addiction.
- We (the medical system) have instructed them to use these to treat their medical symptoms.
- We (the medical system) therefore play an important role in mitigating their risk of addiction or helping to resolve these issues if they arise.
- In many cases, early referral to IBH helps prevent these problems.
• Our cost-benefit analysis of treating them does not make it worthwhile due to time and poor reimbursement.
  ○ The first question to ask is how does the practitioner know this? Or is this a statement that is made in general without data to back it up?
  ○ This should not replace your efforts in your business model (and medical ethics) to address the key patient needs.
• There is a mental health center down the street.
  ○ Yes, but there are many limitations of these systems, and 60% of those will continue to be treated by your PCPs, even if you do refer them.
  ○ Comorbidity is a costly problem (for FQHCs, ACOs, and self-contained systems). Would you prefer to let someone else decrease your cost by treating the mental health condition, or would you prefer to ensure this gets done?
• There are churches and other organizations that can take care of them.
  ○ These are typically volunteer options for supportive care and not for providing self-management skills or medical management to the patient in need.
  ○ Develop relationships with these organizations, they could become a very positive referral sources in smaller communities.
• I don't have enough time in my day to worry about these issues.
  ○ You are spending time on these patients already, whether you realize it or not. There are positive changes in reimbursement upon us.

Appendix 6B.
Calculating a Business Case

A number of variables should be considered when making a thoroughly informed business decision about the financial viability of the integrated behavioral health program you want to launch. A publication[2] produced for the SAMHSA-HRSA Center for Integrated Health Solutions details a business case formula that can be used for a wide range of program implementation paths. We've summarized the details of this formula below.

BUSINESS CASE FORMULA

Cost of Screening **(S)** + Cost of Intervention Services **(I)** + Transition Costs **(T)**

Must Be Less Than or Equal to: $\leq$

Screening Reimbursement **(X)** + Productivity Gains **(P)** + Reimbursement for Treatment **(R)**

$$S+I+T \leq X+P+R$$

Screening (S): Determine the cost of screening by multiplying:
1. How much time is needed to screen each patient?
2. The number of patients who need screening.
3. The salary of the staff doing the screening.

Screening that is built into pre-visit workflows, that devote little if any time for administrative staff or medical assistants to process, decreases the cost of screening—for example having patients complete the Generalized Anxiety Disorder (GAD)-2 screening measure in the waiting room prior to their appointment.

Screening Cost Example
Five (5) minutes for each screening and data entry, 1,200 patients screened a year, by an individual making $25,000 a year equals a screening cost of $1,736 (assuming 1,800 hours worked per year and a fringe rate of 25%).
— Salary including fringe rate is $31,250.
— At 1,800 hours per year that screener is (including fringe) making $17.36 an hour.
— Five (5) minutes screening for 1,200 patients equals 100 hours per year that staff spent screening . . . 100 hours × $17.36 an hour = $1,736.

Intervention (I): Determined by the cost of the person providing the intervention.

Multiply salary (including fringe) **by** Time Needed for the Intervention **by** Patient Volume

Intervention Cost Example
— Salary including fringe rate is $85,000.
— At 1,800 hour per year, the intervention personnel make $47.22 an hour.
— Averages four (4), 30-minute appointments (including documentation). Total of 2 hours spent for each patient.
— Sees 500 unique patients a year.
Multiply 500 patients by 2 hours per patient = 1,000 hours.
— 1,000 hours × $47.22 an hour = $47,220 for the cost of the intervention.

Transition Cost (T): Can include the cost of things like staff training, electronic medical record adaptation, and adapting new workflows or pathways. Transition costs likely will be limited to the first six months of your initial implementation period. Transition cost estimates can be made by summing the costs of:
— Time need for training (e.g., revenue lost by not seeing patients while training);
— Cost of materials and training faculty; and
— The cost, if any, of adapting your electronic medical record templates.

Reimbursement for Screening (X): Reimbursement for screening is variable and subject to federal policy governing Medicare payments, state policy for Medicaid payments, and the unique policy/standard operating procedures of private payers. The good news: there is a positive trend for reimbursement for screening with all major payers. The reimbursement rules must be validated by your clinic/system, given the type of facility you're in, your state and the types of payments you receive. See p. 77 for detailed guidance on funding.

Gains in Productivity (P): Recapturing the cost of lost productivity is a hidden source of funding. Lost productivity happens, for example, when a planned 10-minute appointment turns into a 20-minute appointment as a result of the management of additional depression symptom presentation. In other words, productivity is the number of minutes of primary care provider time that could be made available for other billable appointments. To estimate gains in productivity:
- Observe a sample of patients for one primary care provider over several days;
- Calculate the amount of time for the patients (e.g., 10 minutes for depression) that could have been handled by a BH professional if you had one on site; and
- For your enrolled population, predict how much time could be saved out of a given days panel if the BH piece (e.g., depression) was handled by someone other than your PCP.

Example of Gains in Productivity: Your clinic has 3,500 encounters, all are screened, and 15% screen positive for and would receive care that could be delivered by BH staff (e.g., for depression). This scenario yields 525 (3,500 × .15) appointments where some appointment time could be diverted to a BH staff.

Let's assume that the majority of these 525 patients would receive the extra primary care provider time (10 minutes) for depression that was calculated based on your initial observations. Taking a conservative approach, assume that roughly half (263) are candidates for consultation to your onsite BH person, which will save primary care provider time. If we multiply the 263 candidates by the 10 minutes saved, you get 2,630 minutes that were previously not available. This yields an additional 175 PCP appointments (2,630 minutes divided by 15 [number of minutes for a PCP appointment]). Assuming a reimbursement rate of $135 per PCP appointment this translates into $23,625 in new revenue.

Reimbursement of Interventions (R): Like reimbursement for screening, intervention reimbursement is variable and subject to federal policy governing Medicare payments, state policy for Medicaid payments, and the unique policy/standard operating procedures of private payers. However, there is an increasing trend for payers to reimburse for BH services through direct payment of an appointment or additional per member per month fee in addition to fee-for-service for serving as PCMHs. Bottom line: you'll need to determine what payers are reimbursing what interventions, and what the parameters are (e.g., provider type) that dictate payment. See Appendix 6D for detailed guidance on funding and Table 7.2 in Chapter 7 on Reimbursement Considerations.

Appendix 6C.
Sample Case Study—
Hale Health Center

Let's assume Hale Health Center decides to model Dr. Reims' panel. They decide to observe 100% of Dr. Reims' patient visits for two days. They will determine the burden of illness and also test the workflows necessary to complete screenings and interventions.

As a result of their observation, they find that 65% of Dr. Reims' patients had at least one behavioral health issue that warranted intervention. The observation also revealed that 42% of Dr. Reims' patient visits required more time than the standard appointment interval of 15 minutes. Of these patients, the average time added was 11 minutes. In 80% of the cases where additional time was needed, the extra time was due to behavioral health-related issues that could have been handled by another internal resource.

Among patients needing more time, 40% were covered by Medicaid, 12% by Medicare, and 6% by commercial insurance (primarily BCBS). The remainder were billed using a sliding fee scale. The evidence base suggests 23% of patients who complete an SBIRT screen will be identified as needing an intervention.

Medicaid in the state provides reimbursement for SBIRT at $30.93 for G0396 if a physician does the screening and $26.29 if done by an ancillary provider. Medicare reimburses $29.42 for an SBIRT screening and $57.69 for a screening and intervention.

Hale Health Center assumes that the screening will be built into the front-end work flow in the clinic when patients register and no additional staffing will be added to do the screening. The provider will review the screen as part of the exam and bill accordingly. However, the health center does intend to add a licensed behavioral health professional at an assigned full loaded salary of $81,250. That resource would be shared between two primary care panels and would handle the intervention part of the visit.

The business case per primary care panel would be as follows:

    Panel Size = 1,500

    Annual Encounters = 4,200

    S = No salary cost for SBIRT screening

    I = Allocated salary of $40,625 for the behaviorist (half the total cost allocated to each panel)

    T = Transition costs estimated at 16 hours of total training time for the care team comprised of primary care provider, nurse, and medical assistant. Salary costs are estimated at $72/hr. for a primary care provider, $27.60/hr. for a nurse, and $15.60/hr. for an MA. The total staff time investment would be $1,843.20. They also assumed they would lose revenue of $6,480, assuming 3 visits an hour at an average $135 reimbursement per visit. So T= $8,323.20

Cost then is assumed at $40,625 + $8,323.20 = $48,948.20

On the revenue side, Hale Health Center models the following:

X = SBIRT reimbursement from Medicaid (4,200 encounters × 40% = 1,680 × $24.00 = $40,320). From Medicare it would be (4,200 × 12% = 504 × $29.62 = $14,928.48). Assumes no reimbursement from commercial payers or sliding fee scale. X = $55,248.48.

P = Gains in productivity are calculated based on the number of minutes of primary care provider time that would be freed up and potentially available for another billable visit. If we assume 4,200 encounters and all are screened, 16% will receive an intervention that would result in 672 encounters where a portion of time could be diverted from the provider. A reasonable assumption would be that the majority of these patients are the same ones who are requiring additional time as part of their primary care visit. To be conservative, assume half are candidates for a warm handoff that saves PCP time. We know from the field sampling that Hale Health Center did that the average amount of extra time burden on the PCP was 11 minutes. That would translate into 246 potential patient slots (336 × 11 / 15). If one assumes a reimbursement rate of $135 per PCP visit that would translate to $33,264 of new revenue opportunity.

R = New revenue would be based on the number of SBIRT screens that would be reimbursed for the intervention by the behaviorist working as part of the care team. So we can take our Medicare and Medicaid SBIRT screens (504 + 1,680 = 2,184) and assume 16% result in a brief intervention (349) and then apply the reimbursement rate for an intervention versus a screen. That would translate to 168 × $24.00+ 81 × $29.62 = $8,714.76.

Revenue from integrating screening and intervention would be estimated at $97,227.24

The net business case then would be $97,227.24 − $48,948.20 = $48,279.04 potential above the costs.

This is a hypothetical model and there are obvious flaws and a certain degree of margin for error. For example, it assumes you can capture revenue for all the time redirected from the PCP. The model also does not capture revenue for independent visits by the behaviorists that could be billed and captured. The model does not factor in revenues from tele-health and that would need to be added to the model if reimbursement from payers is available. The model also does not factor in the opportunity gain in revenue from a per member per month fee for care management in Patient-Centered Medical Home Environments.

If Medicaid did not reimburse for SBIRT or intervention, then the net in this example would only be $1,206.01. However, it is still break-even based on Medicare revenue and gains in productivity.

In the end, organizations need to play with their own variables and change its own assumptions to understand the business case. As a result, sensitivity testing can be done for the individual health center environment.

Chapter 6—Business Development

Appendix 6D.
Financing Your Integrated Behavioral Health Service

So everyone thinks this is a great idea and your business case is solid. How is this new service getting funded? A report by the Colorado Health Foundation lists 11 potential fund sources for integrated care, including:
1. Community support/donations/fundraising;
2. Grant funding;
3. Self-pay/sliding scale fee;
4. Billing through current procedural terminology (CPT) codes for BH services;
5. Billing through CPT codes for medical services;
6. Billing through CPT codes for health and behavior codes;
7. Billing screening codes, such as screening, brief intervention and referral to treatment (SBIRT), Patient Health Questionnaire (PHQ)-9, etc.;
8. Internal restructuring of funds;
9. Capitation arrangements (e.g., per screening, per member, per month);
10. Payment arrangements with managed-care organizations; and
11. Joint blending of funds with another organization.

COMMUNITY SUPPORT, GRANT FUNDING, AND SELF-PAY

While some combination of community support, grant funding, and self-pay (i.e., patient pays fees for the service) might be a way to start funding for an IBH program, these funding sources are generally not sustainable. History suggests that even good programs struggle with sustainment as grants run out or the economy changes. Eventually, community support and self-pay are no longer viable options on a system-wide scale. If these seem like the only funding sources for you at this time, we suggest you focus on grant opportunities at the following sources:
- Health Resources and Services Administration (HRSA): www.hrsa.gov
- Substance Abuse and Mental Health Services Administration (SAMHSA): www.samhsa.gov
- Robert Wood Johnson Foundation (RWJF): www.rwjf.org
- Hogg Foundation for Mental Health: www.hogg.utexas.edu
- The California Endowment: www.calendow.org

BILLING THROUGH CODES

At the time of this book's publication, billing for IBH services through various CPT or screening codes was likely to be the most reliable and effective avenue of payment, although still not ideal. Payment through billing codes focuses on the volume of services, not the value of those services, and does not support the alignment of financial and quality outcome incentives across behavioral health and physical systems.

As we mention in Chapter 7, fee-for-service coding is likely to be used as a bridging strategy as we move to global payment reform which revolves around delivering improved health outcomes at lower costs to the payers. Table 7.2 provided various avenues for reimbursement with these codes. Once you've followed the guidance of that table and verified your local and state regulations, consult SAMHSA for specific state billing and financial tools that may be helpful for each state: www.integration.samhsa.gov/financing/billing-tools#Billing. Please be aware that this link is not updated real-time and may not reflect updated state regulations. It is simply a good place for you to start.

Finally, remember to review Figure 6.1, ensuring you follow the step directives on identifying what is viable regarding billing practices. Each state has regulations about what is reimbursable based on site, practice, license, and intervention.

CHAPTER 7
Calculating Value and Revenue Cycles

> **BOTTOM LINE, UP FRONT**
> - Calculating value is an evolving process. Fee-for-service models are dwindling in favor of models that gauge the quality of the care delivered for a specific price rather than how much care is delivered. We are also learning to calculate these fees and values by team rather than individual.
> - Legislative and reimbursement developments make running behavioral health programs more viable and sustainable.
> - You must monitor all your costs and compare these against your revenue.
> - Revenue may be direct (e.g., monies paid to you by a third party) or indirect (i.e., cost offset or cost savings).
> - Use fee schedules and optimal provider types to maximize your reimbursement.
> - Be aware of state and local regulations governing billing for behavioral health and primary care on the same day for the same patient and diagnosis.

Calculating the value of team-based care is a relatively new concept. For some, understanding cost is an important first step in determining value of overall care delivered by both the primary care providers (PCP) and the integrated providers. As the method of care delivery evolves to more team-based services, the need to understand the cost by resources used and value received becomes essential. We contend that patients receive greater value in the form of quality without considerable increase in cost to them or to the payer through a coordinated approach to care. Thus, it is necessary to understand the revenue and cost side, then determine the actual benefits of the team effort.

For example, a PCP may lose time in the exam room dealing with a behavioral health issue that could bring more value to the patient if a behavioral health provider (BHP) team member were involved. The cost of providing integrated care may be lower for the payer, but you will still recoup payment for both the PCP's and the BHP's services. In the end, the patient benefits from the time and skill of both services being delivered and all issues being handled in one place: your medical home. Thus, the dollar cost as well as delivery of care, health outcome, and/or patient satisfaction with care must be considered together in a new approach to achieve value for the patient, the organization, and the healthcare system (the Triple Aim). When done well, integrated care is truly a win-win for patients *and* healthcare systems.

KNOWING YOUR COSTS

The benefits of monitoring your costs include:
- Improves budget, efficiency, and future planning;
- Identifies areas for review and monitoring;
- Identifies areas to streamline practice;
- Promotes development of quality improvement targets;
- Promotes compliance risk assessment;
- Improves negotiation ability in rates and cost setting;
- Provides clarity for pro formas, relative value units (RVUs) and productivity;
- Allows for comparison costs within larger systems and clinics;
- Allows for further program development;
- Promotes cost containment;
- Allows for comparison of reimbursement among payers;
- Allows for comparison of providers; and
- Builds physician compensation models with incentives for quality indicators.

Once you are convinced that costs should be closely monitored (which shouldn't be too difficult), you should answer this important business question: "How much does it cost to see the typical patient?"

The most common answer is, "We don't know."

The real answer is, "There is no such thing as a typical patient."

If you examine the healthcare use of the majority of patients, you are likely to find that they consume a comparable amount of resources, so understanding this cost concept is critical. The main goal is to calculate or even estimate the general cost your organization expends to see a patient. This requires cost accounting, which is essential to determine the costs per patient, per unit of service, or RVUs. (See Appendix 7A for further information on RVUs). These calculations help practices and practice leaders move toward a sustainable delivery of care.

To estimate the cost per patient, follow these steps:

Chapter 7—Calculating Value and Revenue Cycles

Step 1: Identify the visit count using a specific CPT code/type of service for an accounting period of time (monthly, quarterly or annually).

Step 2: Divide the number of visits into the total expenses for that period.

(Typically these steps would not include providers who are owners in the practice, as owners are typically not included in the cost calculations and in smaller practices the owners take what is left at the end of the year to avoid having a corporate tax liability.)

> *To truly build a sustainable integrated care program, we recommend you complete cost calculations and build pro formas (a method of calculating current or projective fiscal results; see Appendix 7G) to create monthly metrics for program accountability and fiscal sustainability.*

Practices can calculate costs per unit of service and break down costs by provider, new versus established patients, diagnosis, departments, service, and/or location (See Appendix 7B). To truly build a sustainable integrated care program, we recommend you complete cost calculations and build pro formas (a method of calculating current or projective fiscal results; see Appendix 7G) to create monthly metrics for program accountability and fiscal sustainability. When sites complete these activities they are able to improve oversight and management of their practice and programs. We recommended you build a chart of accounts (an organization of finances to improve understanding of financial health with regard to specific revenue and expense), control charts (a quality-control strategy to plot and view data overtime compared to the identified control), and monthly reviews of performance within integrated care programs.

UNDERSTANDING REVENUE

Many practices and organizations operate using fee-for-service models. (We include information relevant to reimbursement in the next section, "Current Methods of Revenue Generation.") But since the rise of the Patient-Centered Medical Home (PCMH) model, concomitant developments of Accountable Care Organizations (ACOs), the Patient Protection and Affordable Care Act (PPACA), and other state-level legislation, methods of generating revenue are changing. Alternative payment delivery such as capitated and global payment models may help you facilitate implementation of integrated behavioral healthcare (IBH). In fact, IBH services are one of the product lines that make capitated and global payment models work well. Because these interventions promote better health and prevent disease progression, dollars are saved on patients who would otherwise worsen and require higher (more expensive) clinical services.

Many trusted leaders in integrated care believe such approaches are the way of the future, and states like Colorado[1] and Oregon[2,3] have changed the state health reimbursement legislation to make this a reality. Further, many healthcare programs, organizations, and regulators have developed incentive programs toward value-based payment strategies, including the Robert Wood Johnson Foundation and the Physician Quality Reporting System (PQRS). The PQRS program, which we discussed in the previous chapter, is another example of a value-based payment strategy. These approaches help providers and payers maintain personal accountability and responsibility for how they allocate and provide access to healthcare resources, and facilitate patient engagement in the readily available IBH service.

If value-based payment is the future of our healthcare payment systems, and many believe it is, it will be necessary to develop strategies to manage these payment model changes. We have already mentioned quality programs such as PQRS, universal, global, and capitated payment structures. If you are interested in the direction we are heading for value based care, consider reviewing the proposed 2019 CMS changes related to alternative payment models and merit based incentive payment systems (MIPS) at www.cms.gov/Medicare/Quality-Initiatives-Patient-Assessment-Instruments/Value-Based-Programs/MACRA-MIPS-and-APMs/MACRA-MIPS-and-APMs.html. If you are interested in learning more about these payment options and what the state of Colorado has done, see Section III of this book and this Web site: www.prnewswire.com/news-releases/colorado-health-plans-make-expanded-commitments-to-integrated-care-and-state-innovation-model-300103461.html

CURRENT METHODS OF REVENUE GENERATION

Planning and developing your IBH program may depend on Medicare fee schedules based on provider type and coding and billing options. How you proceed in generating revenue is directly related to your organization type, licensure, state and local laws, and payer policies (See Figure 6.1 in Chapter 6). So as you peruse the following sections, maintain the mindset that these are various options for how to calculate revenue. You may choose one or more of them as you continue developing your business plan and implementing your IBH service.

Consider that IBH suffers from an unfortunate and inaccurate discrimination; it is considered an "extra" service. When establishing a new hospital or practice, few professionals question the importance and value of purchasing radiology equipment, yet the ROI for this may or may not exist. Instead, the organization maintains focus on its relevance to delivering high quality as a result of using this technology. Everything we have learned over the last 40 years in medicine points

Chapter 7—Calculating Value and Revenue Cycles

to the same conclusion with IBH. We know it offers better care than primary care as usual. Similarly, on-boarding IBH should be considered as a necessary service for delivering high quality care, just as radiology and many other expensive aspects of medical care are viewed. Thankfully, IBH is much cheaper and with the right formula may also help you turn a profit.

MAXIMIZE REIMBURSEMENT THROUGH FEE SCHEDULES AND PROVIDER TYPE

One way to plan and develop your integrated care program and service is to examine revenue cycles through reimbursement levels by provider type. It is important to create your fiscal planning reflective of potential direct revenue and reimbursement through billing by provider type and service. Let's take the example of reviewing reimbursement rates through the national Medicare fee schedule (See Table 7.1). By reviewing the table, you will see that the highest reimbursement levels for behavioral health providers are at the doctorate license level. Further, it is important to note that some licenses are not recognized as reimbursed professionals by Medicare.

TABLE 7.1. Medicare Fee Schedule (CMS Medicare Learning Network, September 2013)

Job Title (professional license)	Payment Level
Psychiatrist	100% of physician fee schedule
Clinical Psychologist	100% of physician fee schedule
Nurse Practitioner	85% of physician fee schedule
Physician Assistant	85% of physician fee schedule
Clinical Nurse Specialist	85% of physician fee schedule
Clinical Social Worker	75% of physician fee schedule
Licensed Professional Counselor	Not paid
Licensed Marriage and Family Therapist	Not paid

Irrespective of the model you implement, if you have a considerable revenue stream from Medicare, you may consider hiring licensed professionals who will help you obtain remuneration at the highest rates possible compared to the physician's fee schedule. You also can use this method to identify and refine your provider choice for other payers (private insurance and state Medicaid services). Your ability to tap into one or more of the revenue sources (coding) will depend on the type of licensed professional you hire and Steps 1–3 of the business strategy method listed in Figure 6.1 in Chapter 6.

Since the type of licensed professional will determine which model you select for your program based on what you can bill and code for, let's take a look at codes, beginning with Medicare fee schedules for common codes. Note that some of our colleagues aim for hiring a versatile provider who can support multiple revenue streams. This maximizes their program versatility and flexibility and lowers their risk. This may also maximize their likelihood of a positive return on investment (ROI).

RATES AND CODES FOR BILLING: UNDERSTANDING THE CHALLENGES

Historically, there were restrictions on coverage, number of visits, and copay amounts for mental healthcare services. With the passage of the Mental Health Parity Act (MHPA) of 1996 and the Mental Health Parity and Addiction Equity Act (MHPAEA) of 2008, managing the revenue cycle for mental healthcare has become quite a bit easier. However, there are still complexities and exceptions, which are important for business staff to address (See Appendix 7C). The good news is that since the passing of these acts, mental/behavioral health and physical health copays and services are typically offered with parity/in equal.

Now for the other good news:

- The aforementioned laws require consistent application of benefits for mental health needs similar to medical and surgical coverage. For example, if there is a $20 copay for an office visit for a regular medical visit, the same copay amount applies to a mental health visit.
- PPACA lists one of the eligible health benefits (EHB) as mental health and substance use disorder services, including mental health treatment with counseling and psychotherapy. Thus, healthcare exchange plans require this benefit.

Another item, which complicates billing and reimbursement, is diagnostic coding. If you are new to the mental healthcare world, be aware that the mental health community uses the *Diagnostic and Statistical Manual of Mental Disorders* (DSM) for mental health diagnosis coding. The *DSM,* now in its fifth edition, covers the diagnostic criteria for every mental health disorder. The DSM codes have been "cross-walked" to ICD-9 codes as well as to ICD-10 codes. Ensure your billing and coding staff are knowledgeable about these crosswalks and changes. In addition, ensure your providers are trained on ICD-10 coding and diagnostics. Consider viewing this Medicare Web site: www.cms.gov/Medicare/Coding/ICD10/index.html?redirect=/ICD10

To make reimbursement and direct revenue even more complicated, different insurers and healthcare entities have specific rules and regulations that may benefit or restrict sustainability of integrated care. First, it is significant to note that there are various ways to obtain reimbursement for your IBH services and it is important to diversify. Reimbursement/direct revenue varies based on site type. Center designations include:

- Group practice;

- Federally Qualified Health Center (FQHC);
- Accountable Care Organization (ACO);
- Community Health Center (CHC); and
- Migrant Health Center (MHC), Rural Health Center (RHC), Healthcare for Homeless (HCH), Community-Based Outpatient Clinic (CBOC), Federally Qualified Community Behavioral Health Center (FQCBHC), and Regional Centers.

Site type (with state and federal regulations) then dictates payment model, including prospective payment systems rates, alternative payment methodology (e.g., quality, social determinants, per-member rates), and mixed income. Note that different state and local laws and policy regulations may limit your ability to receive direct revenue reimbursement for services. Table 7.2 lists the relevant reimbursement avenues based on payment determinant and provides considerations to review. Table 7.2 (pages 84–86) also guides you as you develop your business plan despite the restrictions and capabilities for reimbursing IBH in your specific locality.

Once you identify your direct revenue potential, it is essential to understand the CPT and Healthcare Common Procedure Coding System (HCPCS) codes thoroughly. Appendix 7D lists many of the billing codes you could use to capture the IBH workload. Of course, the model you select may influence which ones you use, but your business case analysis (BCA) and business plan will be the final say. In addition, based on your site type and payment model, you may need to develop a list of the modifiers specific to integrated care services (e.g., CMS G Codes and T modifiers).

Another important step is to verify reimbursement rate and coverage per visit. For example, sites can verify coverage through the Medicare Administrative Contractor (MAC). The MAC will issue local carrier determination (LCD) statements of clarification on each code and should be consulted in the plan development phase. In addition, major payers in the market should be consulted for code use, reimbursement levels, and coverage determinations. Many sites verify coverage upon patient check-in for all services provided. Know that one way our colleagues in private-payer settings have succeeded in securing third-party reimbursement for all of these, is to repeatedly bill for them, to meet and communicate directly with these payers to open a dialogue about the changes in the laws, regulations, and the applicable guidelines from the Centers for Medicare & Medicaid Services (CMS).

A great deal of progress can be made through persistence, by politely educating others, and by building relationships . . . or just tenaciously arguing the facts. See the example in Appendix 7E for how to do this with any code. In this case, we selected Health and Behavior Assessment and Intervention (HBAI) Codes in

TABLE 7.2. Reimbursement Considerations

Payment Determinant	Reimbursement Code Types/Categories	Considerations
Medicaid	Health and Behavior Assessment and Intervention (HBAI)	• Requires specific provider license by state regulations • May have different requirements based on site type • Limited frequency; capped in some plans • May have restrictions on same-day funding, depending on site type (i.e., some states note this for FQHCs) • Not all states accept these codes/not "turned on" • States may have restrictions on MH providers only being acknowledged to bill under specified codes
	Psychotherapy	• Requires specific license by state and site type • Limited frequency and/or preauthorization may be required • Not all states allow same-day billing • May require site credentialing
	Prevention and Screening	• Requires specific provider license and designation • Must adhere to defined specifications • Restricted frequency
	Care Coordination/ Chronic Care Management	• Requires specific provider license and designation • Must adhere to defined specifications • Restricted frequency
	Other Specific (Level 2 Office Consult, Prenatal Service Billing, etc)	• Requires specific provider license and designation • Must adhere to defined specifications • Restricted frequency
	Wellness	• Requires specific license and designation • Must adhere to defined specifications • Restricted frequency
Medicare	HBAI	• Requires specific provider license • Limited frequency; capped in some plans • May have restrictions on same-day funding depending on site type (i.e., some states note this for FQHCs) • May require G Codes and modifiers • Medicare advantage plans may have different requirements
	Psychotherapy	• Requires specific provider license type and eligibility • Limited frequency and/or preauthorization may be required • May require copay • May require G Codes and modifiers • Medicare advantage plans may have different requirements
	Wellness	• Requires specific license and designation • Must adhere to defined specifications • May require G Codes and modifiers • Restricted frequency
	Care Coordination/ Chronic Care Management	• Requires specific license and designation • Must adhere to defined specifications • May require G Codes and modifiers • Restricted frequency • Medicare advantage plans may have different requirements

Chapter 7—Calculating Value and Revenue Cycles

	First Step	Next Steps
	• Go to your state's Medicaid Web site and review their requirements.	• Ensure you identify any rules and regulations that pertain to billing and reimbursement procedures for the service type, provider type, and your site type.
	• Go to the main Medicare Web sites to review requirements. • Go to your state's Medicaid Web site and review their requirements and identify any specific references to Medicare billing. • Go to your Medicare Advantage and Supplement plans to review requirements.	• Ensure you identify any rules and regulations that pertain to billing and reimbursement procedures for the service type, provider type, and your site type.

(Continued on next page)

TABLE 7.2. Reimbursement Considerations (continued)

Payment Determinant	Reimbursement Code Types/Categories	Considerations
Medicare (continued)	Prevention and Screening	• Requires specific provider license and designation • Must adhere to defined specifications • May require G Codes and modifiers • Restricted frequency • Medicare advantage plans may have different requirements
	Other Specific (Level 2 Office Consult, Prenatal Service Billing, etc)	• Requires specific provider license and designation • Must adhere to defined specifications • May require G Codes and modifiers • Restricted frequency • Medicare advantage plans may have different requirements
Other Payers	Health and Behavior Assessment and Intervention	• May not offer • May be restricted to specific license • Restricted frequency
	Psychotherapy	• Requires specific provider license type and eligibility • Limited frequency and/or preauthorization may be required • May require additional copay • May require site and provider credentialing
	Wellness	• Requires specific license and designation • Must adhere to defined specifications • Restricted frequency
	Care Coordination/Chronic Care Management	• May not offer • May only be offered by payer • May be restricted to specific license • Must adhere to defined specifications • Restricted frequency
	Prevention and Screening	• May not offer the same as CMS • May be restricted to specific license • Must adhere to defined specifications • Restricted frequency
	Other Specific (Level 2 Office Consult, Prenatal Service Billing, etc)	• May not offer the same as CMS • May be restricted to specific license • Must adhere to defined specifications • Restricted frequency • Explore codes for specific populations to identify other billable services
All Entities	Grants	• Type of services • Type of population • Access to care • Sustainability • Limited scope, breadth, and depth • No guarantee • Limited availability for small group practices

Chapter 7—Calculating Value and Revenue Cycles

First Step	Next Steps
• Go to each insurer's Web site to review billing and practice requirements.	• Ensure you identify any rules and regulations that pertain to billing and reimbursement procedures for the service type, provider type, and your site type.
• Federal (e.g.: grants.gov, SAMHSA/HRSA) • Integration of Care Organizations (e.g., Robert Wood Johnson Foundation, Commonwealth Fund) • Private Insurance Program Grants (e.g., Aetna Foundation) • National Organizations (e.g., American Psychological Association) • State Organizations (e.g., Caring for Colorado Foundation) • Population Specific (e.g., veterans, criminal justice system, military)	• Search for grants to meet your specific population, clinic, and community needs. • Look for grants with which your missions align. • Ensure you are able to pull metrics for monitoring and reporting. • Target reaching populations or providing services that are not already addressed in your reimbursable services.

the next section. For additional information about Medicare and Medicaid reimbursements for IBH, see this Web site: www.integration.samhsa.gov/financing/medicaid-medicare. We encourage all entities, healthcare leaders, and providers to join their local and national associations and state-level committees, build community and stakeholder relationships, and advocate for integrated care sustainability.

It is important to recognize that with all of these challenges to direct revenue, thousands of practices throughout the United States are launching or sustaining their integrated care practices and picking up this book to make them even better! The bottom line is to remember that our larger healthcare system, your system, and bureaucracies in general are not perfect; thus, there will be billing issues. We encourage sites to invest time, energy, and money into billing and coding meetings, training, and personnel related to integrated care sustainability. More specifically, sites may wish to identify a liaison to work with third-party payers and others to negotiate, monitor, and review rejections. Often times, payers may mistakenly reject and approve the same codes on the same or different patients.

In addition, sites need to train front desk, billing and coding staff, as well as providers, on appropriate service procedures. Practice management systems will work fairly well for managing revenue cycles since CPT and ICD codes are used to address encounters and services provided. Training for reception staff, nurses, billing/coding staff, and others is important because administering screening and outcome measures (data), and reporting and billing these may require unique steps that could determine the likelihood of reimbursement. See more details about training in Chapter 10.

You are probably aware of the limitation on use of CPT codes for mental health and HBAI in some states, when an evaluation and management code has already been used for the same diagnosis on the same day. In addition, there are barriers to using mental health codes in healthcare facilities when there are state-contracted behavioral health authorities providing restrictions (e.g., Medicaid partnerships, Medicaid management insurers, and Regional Behavioral Health Authorities). These are barriers to truly integrated care. This fact sheet explains the details and offers additional resources for same-day billing: www.integration.samhsa.gov/financing/Same-Day-Billing-Fact-Sheet-ICN908978.pdf.

Also review your state's regulations for up-to-date information on billing related to your practice site type, funding model, and service. If you are working with Medicaid behavioral health authorities in your state, it's important to identify a liaison to contact and negotiate your site's ability to bill for the additional codes and services they are regulating within reason (e.g., ensure brief intakes, paperwork, interventions, and designation of short-term work with patient/no mental health patient panel development). For additional resources, consider consulting the coding requirements at the following Web sites, which should help your coding and billing staff support your behavioral health providers:

- Health Behavior Assessment and Intervention Codes for individuals, groups, and families (e.g., as used in Primary Care Behavioral Health [PCBH] and Medical Family Therapy [MedFT] Models): www.integration.samhsa.gov/financing/Maine_Health_code.pdf.
- Information for practices relying on private payers (including paying for Care Management Models of IBH): www.integration.samhsa.gov/financing/private-payers
- CPT Codes for Psychotherapy and Psychiatry including revised diagnostic codes (e.g., as used in all models of IBH except Care Management): www.thenationalcouncil.org/topics/coding-behavioral-health-services/
- Free download of book focused on preventative screening for behavioral health in youth (e.g., useful for PCBH and MedFT): www.ncbi.nlm.nih.gov/books/NBK32784/
- Screening, Brief Assessment, Intervention and Treatment codes (e.g., useful for PCBH and MedFT): www.integration.samhsa.gov/clinical-practice/sbirt/financing
- Comprehensive list of tools for billing including same-day billing and other state-specific information (e.g., for all models of IBH): www.integration.samhsa.gov/financing/billing-tools
- U.S. Department of Health and Human Services resources on chronic care management (e.g., for Care Management Model) www.cms.gov/Outreach-and-Education/Medicare-Learning-Network-MLN/MLNProducts/Downloads/ChronicCareManagement.pdf

Overall, to sustain your program with regard to the Triple Aim, you must ensure appropriate, timely, and relevant documentation of the services you code and bill. We include specific guidance to help you document the codes you are billing. We encourage you to use the information in Appendix 7F and Table 7.2, as well as your PMS, EHR, etc., to develop auditing tools that address:

- Timeliness of completion.
- Justification of services.
- Relevancy/consistency with which evidence-based interventions are delivered and are appropriate given the patient's symptoms, diagnosis and plan.
- Whether or not the documentation meets the appropriate payer criteria for payment.
- Patient's response to care.
- Patient satisfaction data.
- Care coordination with PCP and the care team.
- Relevant goals to overall health and wellness.

- Care team management.

These factors drive quality of care, successful payment, positive patient experience, and with enough patients over time, a lower overall cost to payers.

CALCULATING THE ROI

Skepticism about integrated care has arisen predominantly in systems that rely entirely on fee-for-service payment models. In these circles, there is some worry among leaders that if their patients become healthier due to enhanced services, such as integrated behavioral health, and therefore decrease their use of primary care services, the healthcare providers will experience reduced income. This is not true. If each of your PCPs carries 2000 patients on his or her panel, improving the health of this panel with concomitant decreases in their annual primary care use enables the PCP to increase the size of his or her panel or the parent organization's market share. This means growth for the organization that employs these PCPs. While this sounds simple at a macro level, the details of accomplishing it requires some work, beginning with how you calculate a return on investment (ROI).

IBH activities should be monitored with the ability to pull those activities out of the rest of the primary care service as part of quality assurance to determine if the collection process is working well. We suggest developing a set of administrative key performance indicators (KPIs) for your integrated care service that are consistent with your business goals. Benchmark KPIs might include:

- Days in Receivables outstanding—30 days or less. This is average daily charges over a long period of time. For example, 6 to 12 months divided into the current outstanding accounts receivable.
- Percentage over 120 days aging—10% or less. This is simply pulled from the aged trial balance printed regularly in your PMS dashboard.
- Net collection percentage—95% to 98%. This is the actual dollars eligible for collections, minus contractual allowances, which is effectively bad debt.

There may be other KPIs that are important for your unique circumstance. The key is to set up your system to track patients who meet your integrated treatment program requirements. This tracking can be based on diagnosis (a good way to identify the current patient population) or by PCP or BHP. For example, if you operate a Care Management program for depression, you want to be able to identify those individuals if they have seen the behavioral health care facilitator, and evaluate the administrative KPIs on those patients.

Don't overlook that patients may have a mental health diagnosis listed as second or third on their problem/diagnosis list with a medical diagnosis as primary. The effect the second or third diagnosis has on the patient outcome will be important to monitor. It is possible that although your PCPs are treating a gen-

TABLE 7.3. The Cost of Co-occurring Mental Health Disorders and Chronic Conditions

	PPPY Cost—Those Without MH Condition	PPPY Cost—Those with MH Condition	The Cost of Co-occurring Conditions
Heart Condition	$4,697	$6,919	$2,222
High Blood Pressure	$3,481	$5,492	$2,011
Asthma	$2,908	$4,028	$1,120
Diabetes	$4,172	$5,559	$1387

Original source data has been integrated.[4]

eral health condition, the patient has been treated in the past for a mental health diagnosis, but is not currently engaged in mental health treatment. Alternatively, the patient may be engaged in treatments delivered by your PCPs (i.e., medication management), and now that you've brought a BHP on board, he or she can deliver additional evidence-based interventions that you can bill for in addition to the PCP's treatments.

Taken together, better, more comprehensive care is delivered and billed for with IBH on board. For example, the cost of treating a chronic health condition without treating the co-occurring mental health condition costs more (See Table 7.3) according to Health and Human Services data from 2002–2003.[4] These are opportunities to excel clinically and in business terms, particularly through collaboration with your payers, who will greatly appreciate the value of these data and the services you provide.

SAMPLE ROI CALCULATIONS

So what's the bottom line? If a single staff member, such as a clinical psychologist, is added, the direct cost including benefits could be in the area of $80,000. If reimbursement is $70 per visit based on a 99213 or 90846 and screening, this BHP would have to see approximately 1100 visits to break even. If practice overhead of 50% is applied to salary, the visit number increases to 1700. If we look back at the HBAI codes and note about $20 per 15-minute Medicare allowance (for a randomly selected region in the southern United States), moving to a full hour of HBAI work is greater than the $70 per-visit calculated through the CPT and screening services by $10 or more. If we look at an annual total of 2080 hours paid at the hourly rate for a BHP who is a clinical psychologist (about $40), any hour worked over 50% of total will yield a nice return.

Also as previously mentioned, there will be offset gains. Since the PCP has freed up time through the team model, he or she may see one more patient per day at current Medicare allowable amounts. This means the practice gains $20,000 with no real cost associated with the visit. Note that we found that on average, PCPs receive 56 minutes back, and the clinic saves an average of 18 minutes for every patient referred to the BHP (PCBH Model[5]). The combination of the BHP services, freeing up time for the PCP, and efficient billing practices will yield substantial financial benefits to the practice. For example, one pediatric IBH program concluded that PCPs spent 2 fewer minutes for every patient seen on a day when a BHP was present. PCPs also saw 40% more patients on days when the BHP was providing services. The practice was able to collect $1,142 more revenue on days when the BHP was present (PCBH Model)[5].

Let's go one step further: When we insert the BHP into the PCP workflow so the new emphasis is on managing chronic diseases and the patient's care (using any of these models alone or in combination [PCBH, MedFT, Care Management]), we are pursuing the Triple Aim objective. We improve the quality of patient care through improved coordination of the individual care, compliance with the overall care plan, and reduction of issues that may lead to admission, re-admission, or unnecessary use of the emergency department.

For example, the CMS created codes for management of chronic diseases and transition from a hospital stay to the next step(s) in treatment. As such, you may receive additional payment based on quality metrics and healthcare cost reduction. Consider this example:

After hospital discharge, the chronic care patient (e.g., diabetes, renal failure) benefits from contact by the care manager or care facilitator because this staff member conducts medication reconciliation and discusses risks of falls and related matters in the patient's home and by checking the status of key clinical indicators. The transition care approach ensures the patient is seen within 7 (high—90496) or 14 (moderate—90495) days of discharge from the hospital. In addition, staff should visit the patient's home or at the very least follow up with a series of phone calls. In both examples related to chronic diseases, a behavioral health staff member, such as a nurse, may be involved and offer the right level of service needed for the patient and for the medical home team.

> ***Through formal management procedures such as Lean 6 Sigma, control charts, Gantt charts, Re-Aim, PDSA, workflows, and pro forma, the way you measure program metrics (Chapter 8), and the way you understand your KPIs (earlier in this chapter), you can achieve success where some have fallen short.***

The behavioral health personnel will be part of the team that reaches out to the patient and/or family. This may not result in direct revenue, but can be a key factor in the review of the project plan and the ROI for the positions. It also offsets costs because the PCP is not reaching out, but is spending billable hours performing tasks that are unique to the PCP skill set (which no one else can do) or that lead to high reimbursements from payers per task.

Remember, this is one of the most common and detrimental mistakes in launching IBH programs: poor model fidelity and not utilizing the service to its full capacity.[6,7] Through formal management procedures such as Lean 6 Sigma, control charts, Gantt charts, Re-Aim, PDSA, workflows, and pro forma, the way you measure program metrics (Chapter 8), and the way you understand your KPIs (earlier in this chapter), you can achieve success where some have fallen short. If you are interested in learning various management strategies for successful monitoring and improvement, we encourage you to seek independent and formalized management training, executive leadership training, and/or continuing education through the resources listed in the Ongoing Training section of Chapter 10.

A DEEPER DIVE INTO ROI

To build a sustainable integrated care program, organizations must identify the ROI. ROI formulas are important for all healthcare entities that are looking toward or evaluating the IBH programs and who have a level of reimbursement, whether it is through direct billing, grants, or indirect revenues. Medical homes are strongly encouraged to evaluate their IBH programs from both an ROI and cost-savings approach.

There are multiple ways to calculate ROI in integrated healthcare. It is important for organizations to familiarize themselves with the various analyses for quality improvement. We will start with a simple ROI formula and demonstrate how to use it within integrated care.

$$\text{ROI:} \frac{\text{gain from program} - \text{cost of program}}{\text{cost of program}} \times 100 = \text{percent of ROI}$$

This formula demonstrates the dollars spent on a program versus dollars earned from the program. The monies gained are the direct income generated by direct payment for completed/billed IBH services. The cost of the program is the direct employee costs for an IBH provider. Often, organizations may wish to add the direct monies earned by the PCP being able to see additional patients per day, or "upcode" from the addition of an IBH provider (see pro forma examples in Appendix 7G). When using pro formas, don't forget that our examples in the Appendices are general. Each pro forma you run will be unique to the BHP due to his/her specific salary, benefits, and reimbursement strategy. Note that pro formas will vary considerably and each one involves any number of different assumptions. As you change these assumptions and your other parameters, the projected results change accordingly. We encourage you to be persistent in developing these until you have the outcomes you want. Appendix 7H offers formulas and brief discussions of additional ROI types, such as cost savings and cost offset. Using more than one type of ROI helps you quantify the multiple benefits to IBH. It also helps you analyze your healthcare services similarly to how our changing healthcare system will evaluate you in the future.

References

1. Colorado Innovation Model. http://www.colorado.gov/healthinnovation
2. Oregon Primary Care Transformation Initiative. http://www.oregon.gov/oha/legactivity/SB%20231%20(PC%20transformation)%20one-pager%201.21.15.pdf
3. Oregon Coordinated Care Organizations (CCOs). http://cco.health.oregon.gov/Pages/Home.aspx
4. U.S. Dept of HHS the 2002 and 2003 MEPS. AHRQ as cited in Petterson et al. "Why there must be room for mental health in the medical home (Graham Center One-Pager); Hertz RP, Baker CL. The impact of mental disorders on work. *Pfizer Outcomes Research*. Publication No P0002981. Pfizer; 2002.
5. Gouge N, Polaha J. Integration can work! Demonstrating cost effectiveness and marketing it in the real world. Paper presented at the annual meeting of the Collaborative Family Healthcare Association, 2013, Denver, CO.
6. *IHI 90-Day R&D Project Final Summary Report: Integrating Behavioral Health and Primary Care*. Cambridge, MA: Institute for Healthcare Improvement; March 2014. Available at www.ihi.org.
7. Scharf DM, Eberhart NK, Hackbarth NS, et al. *Evaluation of the SAMHSA Primary and Behavioral Health Care Integration (PBHCI) Grant Program: Final Report (Task 13)*. Santa Monica, CA: RAND Corporation; 2014. http://www.rand.org/pubs/research_reports/RR546.html. Accessed April 24, 2015.

Appendix 7A.
Relative Value Unit

RVUs are the national standard for measuring the base unit of provider work, productivity, budgeting, expenses, and cost benchmarking. There are two major ways to understand and use relative value units (RVUs) in healthcare to represent the cost of providing a service: 1) CMS calculations for each CPT/HCPCS code (i.e., 90832) or service calculations, and 2) site-specific calculations/practice expenses. RVU calculations are important for healthcare practices because the help with identifying the compensation and cost of a service. The three main types of RVUs are:

1. Provider work RVUs (wRVUs) which may include relative level of time, technical skill, effort, and intensity of a service for which CMS provides a RVU to each associated CPT code, or reimbursable amounts and costs of provider salary, benefits, and payroll tax;
2. Practice expense RVUs (peRVUs) includes all of the direct (non-clinical and non-provider clinical labor) and indirect costs (building space, equipment, supplies) for running a practice; and
3. Malpractice overhead/professional liability RVUs (mpRVUs) includes the costs of professional liability and insurance.

RVUs are not monetary values; rather, they represent relative amount of provider work, resources, and expertise needed to provide a specific service. It is important to identify the RVU needs and calculations for your practice to assist with fiscal sustainability of the practice, program, and providers. Many provider salaries are determined by the amount of RVUs a provider is able to produce in a given year.

To be most efficient, healthcare practices must research the CMS Resource Based RVUs (RBRVU) and/or utilize Geographic Practice Cost Index (GPCI) for accurate measurement. Healthcare practices can identify the RVUs for individual CPT/HCPCS codes by accessing the Centers for Medicare and Medicaid Services website via the Physician Fee Schedule Look-Up Tool, www.cms.gov/apps/physician-fee-schedule/overview.aspx. In addition, the healthcare practice reimbursement modality is essential to consider for fiscal sustainability. In some practices, panel size with risk adjustment may be more defining. Although RVUs are essential to practice management, quality, efficiency, effectiveness, and satisfaction must always be held in highest value.

An example of using RVUs to support fiscal sustainability is completing site-specific RVU calculations to gauge productivity. There are many different productivity calculations. One way to gauge productivity is by deriving a productivity ratio through the equation: % provider revenue / % provider RVU (expenses) = productivity ratio. The percentage of provider revenue (based on the total revenue) is divided by the RVU expenses (percentage may include wRVU, peRVU, and mpRVU based on total expenses) to get the provider's percent of the total RVUs.

As an example, there are 10 providers at a clinic (all other things remaining equal). Dr. Shneebley is one who responsible for $100,000 in revenue out of a total of $1 million in practice revenue, which results in 10% provider revenue of the total practice revenue. If his provider RVU is at 10%, then he has a 1:1 ratio, meeting productivity standards. If his revenue is lower at $50,000 out of $1 million (as 10% of the providers), then his ratio is .5 to 1, adding $50,000 in cost. Using these calculations and RVUs allows healthcare practices and managers to become more fiscally minded regarding practice and performance management.

The following are RVU formulas that many healthcare entities use:
- (% provider revenue) / (% provider RVU (expenses)) = productivity ratio
- (wRVU x wGPCI) + (peRVU x peGPCI) + (mpRVU x mpGPCI) = RVU formula for any CPT code
- (Sum of total expenses) / (Sum of total RVUs) = Cost per RVU

Appendix 7B.
Sustainable Integrated Care Programs Depend on Frequently Calculating Costs

CALCULATING COSTS PER UNIT

Step 1: Identify unit/type of service. Identify unit based on what is relevant for your practice (e.g., service time in 15-minute increments, claims, CPT/HCPCS visits, types of patients, etc.).

Step 2: Identify the number of units of service provided in a designated time period (e.g., monthly, quarterly, yearly).

Step 3: Identify direct costs (expenses easily relatable to the service/unit). For example, provider and support staff salaries/benefits cycle time (per-cycle time related to service or formulated based on minutes of salary/benefits) is the length of time a patient may be engaged, from entering site to completion of service/leaving site, supplies, and other resources consumed during service. Be careful and detailed.

Step 4: Identify indirect costs (expenses shared by more than one area of practice), such as larger operational, administrative, and facility costs (typically taking a percentage). This may be calculated through percentages relative to providers, services, square footage, etc.

Step 5: Identify depreciation. Many sites will review depreciation so they do not overlook long-term expenses for planning.

Step 6: Identify the full cost of the unit of service by adding the costs from Steps 3, 4, and 5.

Appendix 7C. Mental Health Parity and Addiction Equity Act (MHPAEA) Information

MHPAEA Full Information:	- www.cms.gov/CCIIO/Programs-and-Initiatives/Other-Insurance-Protections/mhpaea_factsheet.html#Summary - www.samhsa.gov/health-financing/implementation-mental-health-parity-addiction-equity-act
MHPAEA Exceptions Include:	- Employers with 50 or fewer employees need not meet the terms of the MHPAEA. That sounds easy, but each state may define the small employer at 100 employees due to the requirements of the PPACA. - There must be medical necessity (a term variably defined by each payer). - There may be a need for authorization for coverage if there is preauthorization required for medical or surgical services. - An insurance plan may be exempt if the cost of inclusion of these benefits increases their cost of providing mental healthcare by greater than 2% for one year. - State and local government plans that are self-insured may opt-out of the requirements if they take some administrative steps. See this Web site for further information: www.dol.gov/ebsa/faqs/faq-aca17.html - The MHPAEA does NOT apply to retiree-only health plans. - If an employer plan did not offer mental health coverage in the past they may be exempt regardless of the number of employees.

Appendix 7D.
Billing Codes

H&B CPT Code	Description of Documentation
96150: Initial Assessment	• Onset and history of initial diagnosis of physical illness • Clear rational for H&B assessment • Assessment outcome • Mental status and document patient's ability to understand directions and interventions (patient must have cognitive capacity) • Goals and expected duration of intervention • Length of time of assessment and date • Identification of biopsychosocial factors affecting condition/treatment • Ensure this assessment does not duplicate other assessment completed • Ensure physician has documented need for this assessment
96151: Re-Assessment	• Significant change in mental or medical status requiring assessment; change cannot be due to mental health illness • Date of change in status requiring re-assessment • Clear rationale for re-assessment • Clear indication of precipitating event • Length of time of re-assessment and date • Re-assessment does not need to be completed by same provider who completed initial • Ensure physician has documented need • Ensure all requirements from 96150 above are met/documented
96152: Follow up 96153: Group	• Length of visit and date • Mental status and document patient's ability to understand directions and interventions (patient must have cognitive capacity) • Clearly defined intervention addressing biopsychosocial concerns with amelioration of medical/physical illness concerns/improving physiological functioning, disease status, and health and wellbeing • Goals of intervention • Identification of how intervention improves adherence to medical plan • Response to intervention • Rationale for frequency and duration of services • Consultations

(Continued on next page)

H&B CPT Code	Description of Documentation
96154: Intervention with Family and Patient Family is defined as: • Primary/immediate family • Extended family • Caregiver • Guardian • Health care proxy	• Must be reasonable and necessary to include patient and family care • Family must directly participate in patient's care • Family involvement is necessary to address the biopsychosocial factors and assist with adherence to medical plan • Ensure all requirements from 96152 above are met/documented
96155: Intervention with Family Without Patient	• Ensure all requirements from 96154 and 96152 above are met/documented

PSYCHOTHERAPY CPT CODE BASICS

Psychotherapy CPT Code	Description of Documentation
90791: Initial Assessment	• Identification of mental health or substance use problem • Treatment planning • Identification of measurable goals • Justification of services • Functional impairment • Referral question
90832: 30-minute session (16–37 minutes) 90834: 45-minute session (38–52 minutes) 90837: 60-minute session (53+ minutes; not reimbursed across all payers; may be crisis limited)	• Start and stop times and date • Length of face-to-face minutes • Justification of treatment • Mental status • Formal and informal assessment • Identification of specific interventions (evidence-based) and overall efficacy • Patient's response to treatment • Progress made toward mental health measureable goals/objectives • Clinical decision making • Functional status and current level of symptoms • Prognosis and adherence • Risk • Plan and referrals • Consultations
Group	• Summary of group's behavioral health goals and purpose • Primary focus of patient in group interaction and involvement • Group relevancy to patient's treatment plan and needs • Total number of patients in group • Length of group times; start and stop time; date

Appendix 7E.
Educating Your Payers

If you already have an IBH program (i.e., if you are running the PCBH or medical family therapy models) AND you accept not getting reimbursed for HBAI codes as the cost of doing business (due to the benefits it has on the staff and patients), then well done, you are committed to integrated care.

Consider following the steps below to begin the process of resolving a reimbursement problem—in this example, HBAI codes. In some states, payers won't reimburse for HBAI codes, as they follow Medicare schedules, which vary. Some state Medicare agencies turn these "on or off." The following resource is the only consistently updated source for HBAI and SBIRT billing information that we know of. We recommend while developing your program, you verify with your state if these codes are listed on your state's fee schedule: my.ireta.org/sbirt-reimbursement-map.

Once you decide you'd like to do something about this, there are two primary steps you can take that could lead to reimbursement for HBAI codes.

STEP 1. PREPARE YOUR DATA

Schedule a meeting with your finance management, clinic/system leadership; then prepare all of your data so you can present them. Use the figures listed in Table 6.1 and Table 7.3, and the case examples in Section III to assist with this task. These are very powerful data with which you can educate them about how paying now subsequently will save them money across the population.

Be sure everyone has a clear idea of why this is important from a health perspective and the potential impact on cost over time for the third-party payer. If possible, pull your own data on patients prior to receiving services under the HBAI codes and services after these interventions. If there are data showing decreased referral to specialists, decreased hospitalization or re-hospitalization, decreased Emergency Department use, increased use of preventive services (e.g., well baby visits), or improved health biomarkers (e.g., Hemoglobin A1c within normal limits), these data should be used for future discussions with third-party payers.

There also may be value in talking with payers in other states and finding out why it was important for them to pay for services that fall under these codes. What is important to one payer is likely to be important to other payers and you can use that information to help make your argument for reimbursement when you go to Step Two.

STEP 2. MEET WITH YOUR PAYERS

Schedule a meeting with the payers. Prior to the meeting, designate a primary speaker who will present an argument about why HBAI codes should be reimbursed (based on data and discussions from Step 1). Ask other finance management, administrative, and clinic leadership subject matter experts to attend this meeting to assist with questions that fall outside of the primary speaker's area of expertise.

Developing relationships with the payers and helping them learn the potential benefits of HBAI reimbursement, not only within your system, but in other systems within the state, may be instrumental in making progress in your own system being reimbursed or in payer statewide payment changes. We know that systems/providers have secured buy-in and reimbursement in some states by a similar process.

In summary, for those relying at least partially on private payers, first see if your state reimburses HBAI codes. If the answer is yes, this makes your next set of development decisions easier. If not, review these Web sites and ensure you verify this information, as policies change rapidly (and surreptitiously . . . can you believe it?):

- **Same Day Billing:** www.integration.samhsa.gov/financing/Same-Day-Billing-Fact-Sheet-ICN908978.pdf
- **State Use of HBAI Codes:** www.integration.samhsa.gov/images/res/Map_of_Available_HBAI_CPT_Codes1.pdf
- **Financing of Behavioral Health Services:** www.integration.samhsa.gov/financing

Appendix 7F. Documentation

You cannot ensure reimbursement without quality efforts related to ensuring evidence-based interventions, care, and documentation of such. When basics are not regulated and monitored, a thorough chart audit may result in significant fines and payback of reimbursement. In integrated behavioral health (IBH), documentation must balance the needs of many. Documentation is an essential and vital tool of health care delivery and risk management.

An old adage about documentation is to consider charting with an anxious patient on one shoulder, a highly aggressive lawyer and auditor on the other, and being surrounded by the entire care team. BHPs must learn documentation that is succinct, accurate, timely, and useful. Documentation shares the burden of balancing the information and needs of many, while being a primary tool for communication of continuity of care.

For truly integrated care, behavioral health providers (BHPs) must document in a shared medical record. BHPs must be trained regarding documentation within the medical record, best practice related to documentation, payer requirements, and coding requirements. In addition, they must learn the lens of documenting what is essential and relevant for the patient, for the care team, and for the future.

IBH providers must receive training on appropriate expectations for documentation content and timeliness. Documentation includes consultation responses, follow-up, phone contact, face-to-face contact, and progress notes. In many medical homes, BHPs are required to update the medical record with regard to various EHR medical standardization review and share the responsibility of updating the master problem list and medication list. It is important BHPs use their expertise in diagnostics to ensure diagnosis reconciliation of charts and to review mental health conditions present. Any change to the medical record master lists should have a notation about the reason for the change and evidence (history, report, document or care reference) to support.

For many, shared care goals are included in the EHR and must be monitored with each visit. Documentation should be completed in the medical record for IBH. Many medical homes have a mechanism to automatically share all updated documentation of a patient record with the care team. This tool can be used to ensure the team reviews and signs off on the episode of care. In addition, dependent on your level of integration and confidentiality legalities, BHPs may need to document in a separate secure chart. Separate documentation is a barrier for truly informed and integrated care. It is important for practices to review this workflow to determine if there is flexibility to build a higher level of integration within the system.

IBH documentation differs from traditional mental health documentation. In integrated care it is important to recognize the documentation must negotiate care team review. Documentation should be general, pertinent to the patient's health and wellness and continuity of care, relevant and understandable to the patient and care team, and limited related to sensitive information. Providers should not document topics such as specifics to past traumas, counter transference or transference, dream analysis, and quotes, which are unrelated to symptomatology and health status. In addition, reportable events must be managed following the medical center guidelines and workflows related to documentation and ethics.

WORKFLOW, AUDITING, AND TRAINING

It is the responsibility of integrated care managers to develop workflows, auditing tools, and trainings related to integrated care documentation. Documentation review is an essential part of quality assurance, improvement, and compliance standards. It is also the responsibility of the organization to ensure documentation is aligned with standard practice, organizational, accreditation, state, federal, professional practice, and payer policies and procedures.

Workflows and reviews are best when developed accordingly and adaptable to be operationalized and applied. They should provide clear guidance and be reviewed annually. Further, it is important for management to consider building a structured auditing tool related to ensuring compliant and relevant documentation. Use CPT coding for program quality assurance and for pro forma monitoring. Monitor regarding documentation timeliness on completion and monitor with the billing department to ensure successful reimbursement.

ALIGNING WITH CPT CODING

Medical necessity is required for all services provided. Medical necessity is defined as the existence of evidence for therapeutic decision making toward services that are reasonable and necessary for the diagnosis and treatment of an illness or injury, to improve functioning. Medical necessity informs type and level of service.

For IBH providers, health behavior and assessment intervention, psychotherapy, and wellness codes are used most frequently. Below are recommendations related to documentation to align with CPT coding.

Health Behavior and Assessment Intervention Codes (HBAI or H&B Codes):

1. Review Appendix 7D (specifically HBAI codes).
2. Primary medical diagnosis (non-DSM code).

3. Identification of biological, psychophysiological, behavioral, or social factors affecting the medical treatment.
4. Prevention, treatment, or management of physical health/medical diagnosis.
5. Focus on biopsychosocial factors.
6. Assessment may include: interviews, mental status, measureable progress, health-oriented questionnaires, onset of illness, and outcome measurement of specific interventions.
7. Examples of treatment intervention include: improving adherence to medical treatment, symptom management, health-promoting behaviors, and targeting reduction of health risk-taking behaviors.
8. Bill in 15-minute increments; limited to 4 units regardless of intervention needed.
9. Review payer-specific requirements; many insurance plans have yearly H&B reimbursable limits.
10. Review licensure, state, and federal regulations to ensure reimbursement eligibility (review Figure 6.1).

Psychotherapy Coding

1. Review Appendix 7D (specifically psychotherapy CPT codes).
2. Primary mental health or substance use/abuse concern (DSM 5/ICD 10 code).
3. Identification of biological, psychophysiological, behavioral, or social factors affecting the medical treatment.
4. Prevention, treatment, or management of mental health and substance abuse conditions and symptomatology affecting health and functioning.
5. Assessment may include: interviews, mental status, measureable progress, questionnaires, onset of illness, and outcome measurement of specific interventions.
6. Examples of treatment interventions include: improving adherence to treatment, symptom management, health-promoting behaviors, and targeting mitigation of symptoms and self-management.
7. Billed correlated to intervention, face-to-face time.
8. Review payer-specific requirements; many insurance plans have yearly reimbursable limits and preauthorization requirements.
9. Review licensure, state and federal regulations to ensure reimbursement eligibility (review Figure 6.1).
10. Name the documentation in terms of progress notes rather than psychotherapy notes, which are defined differently by HIPPA.

Appendix 7G.
Pro Forma

Pro Forma is a method of calculating current or projective fiscal results to create financial metrics for program accountability and fiscal sustainability. Through this planning improvement strategy, organizations can improve control, management, and planning of programs. Further, organizations can use pro formas to demonstrate sustainability and provide analysis for investment, credit, and program growth adjustment. Building pro formas involves identifying the payer mix, reimbursement rates, prospective program costs, and needed revenue generation. Monitoring through pro formas involves comparisons to profit/loss projections, balance sheets, revenue generation, and to similar programs and organizations.

Below are examples of pro formas based on integrated care at various centers (general integrated care pro forma, FQHC wrap-around PPS rate/no same-day visit pro forma, and group practice mixed payer pro forma). Each of the pro forma examples below is based on a conservative effort of behavioral health provider utilization. Many behavioral health providers average double or slightly less than double—it depends on practice management, clinic culture and expectation of care delivery; the IBH model selected; and training. It is essential that clinics recognize the importance of these elements when integrating.

Sample Pro Formas

Integrated Behavioral Health Provider Pro Forma Example

	Identify how many BH visits per year	X,XXX		
	Identify estimate of how many will be reimbursed	XX%		
			XXXXX	Total Number of Visits Reimbursed
Consider listing each insurance separately and actual reimbursement rate	Est. reimb per Psychotherapy code visit	$XX	XXXXX	Number of visits reimbursed
	SBIRT/Brief Screening	$XX	XXX	Number of visits reimbursed
	Est. reimb per HBAI code visit	$XX	XXX.X	Number of visits reimbursed
	Total Visits		XXXXX	Total Number of Visits Reimbursed
			XXXXXX	

Chapter 7—Calculating Value and Revenue Cycles

Variable 1: Indirect Revenue *Consider listing each type separately for tracking and productivity. This will go into the job description and monitoring*	Contribution Margin/Net	XXX	(conservative 2 patients per day offset or increase in year for Medical Provider: dual visit, optimal coding, group visit, increased access)	
		$XX.00 per visit		
		$XXXX.00	$XXXX.00	
	Doctorate Level Net Revenue		**$XXXXX.00**	From reimburseables above
	Masters Net Revenue (usually pays between 10 and 20% less for private payers; 25% less for Medicare)		**$XXXXX.00**	May be different; dependent on license and reimbursement rate
Variable 2: Other forms of Revenue	Grant funding	$X,000		
List potential grants	Total Net Revenue		**$XXXXX.00**	
Salary of your BHP	Doctorate Level (1.0 FTE)	$XX,000		
Benefits of your BHP	Benefits	$XX,000		
	Total compensation	$XXX,000		
Salary of your BHP	Masters Level (1.0 FTE)	$XX,000		
Benefits of your BHP	Benefits	$XX,000		
	Total compensation	$XXX,000		
Additional benefits	CME	$X,000		
	Laptops	$X,000		
Personnel or program expenses	Coding & billing expense	$XX,000		
	Total Expenses Doctorate Level		$XX,000	
	Total Expenses Masters Level		$XX,000	
	Doctorate Level BHP Revenue		**$XX,000**	
	Masters Level BHP Revenue		**$XX,000**	

General Integrated Behavioral Health Provider Pro Forma Example

	Annual Visits per BHP	2,750	
	Reimbursable visits	75%	
			2,062.50
	Est. reimb per Psychotherapy code visit	$65.00	1032
	SBIRT/Brief Screening	$25.00	515
	Est. reimb per HBAI code visit	$20.00	515
	Total Visits		2062
			$90,255
Variable 1	Contribution Margin/Net	400	(conservative 2 patients per day offset or increase in year for Medical Provider: dual visit, optimal coding, group visit, increased access)
		$85.00 per visit	
		$34,000	$34,000
	Doctorate Level Net Revenue		$124,255
	Masters Net Revenue (usually pays between 10 and 20% less for private payers; 25% less for Medicare; these calculations based on 85% of physician fee schedule)	$124,255	$105,617
Variable 2	Grant funding	5,000	
	Total Net Doctorate Level Revenue		**$129,255**
	Total Net Masters Level Revenue		**$110,617**
	Doctorate Level (1.0 FTE)	80,000	
	Benefits	20,000	
	Total compensation	100,000	
	Masters Level (1.0 FTE)	65,000	
	Benefits	16,250	
	Total compensation	81,250	
	CME	1,750	
	Laptops	1,500	
	Coding & billing expense	5,816	
	Total Expenses Doctorate Level		109,066
	Total Expenses Masters Level		90,316
	Doctorate Level BHP Revenue		**$20,189**
	Masters Level BHP Revenue		**$20,300**

Integrated Behavioral Health Provider Pro Forma Example for FQHC with Wrap-Around Funding PPS Rate $200.00 Visit, No Same-Day Billing Reimbursement

	Annual CMS Visits per provider	2,750	
	Reimbursable visits (50% are same-day)	50%	
			1,375.00
	CMS Psychotherapy code visit	$200.00	$687.00
	Private Insurer	$50.00	$338.00
	CMS HBAI code visit	$200.00	$350.00
	Total Visits		1375
			$224,300
Variable 1	Contribution Margin/Net	150	(conservative 2 patients per week offset or increase in year for PCP: dual visit, upcoding, group visit, increased access)
	Per-Visit Reimbursement	$200.00	
		$30,000	$30,000
	BHP Level Net Revenue		**$254,300**
Variable 2	Grant funding	5,000	
	50 Grant Funded Visits (population specific)	$50.00	
	Total Net Revenue		**$259,300**
	Doctorate Level BHP (1.0 FTE)	$80,000.00	
	Benefits	$20,000.00	
	Total compensation	$100,000.00	
	Masters Level BHP (1.0 FTE)	$65,000.00	
	Benefits	$16,250.00	
	Total compensation	$81,250.00	
	CME	$1,750.00	
	Laptops	$1,500.00	
	Coding & Billing Expense	$11,668.50	
	Total Expenses Doctorate Level		$114,918.50
	Total Expenses Masters Level		$96,168.50
	Doctorate Level BHP Revenue		**$144,381.00**
	Masters Level BHP Revenue		**$163,131.00**

Group Practice Mixed Payor Pro Forma Example

	Annual Visits per BHP	3,000	
	Considering 1 BHP to 1 Medical Providers		
	Reimbursable Visits	85%	
	(requires paneling on all insurances)		2,550.00
	Medicaid Psychotherapy code visit	$55.00	650
	Medicare Psychotherapy code visit	$62.00	800
	Medicaid HBAI code visit	$21.00	250
	Medicare HBAI code visit	$21.00	350
	Private Insurer Psychotherapy code visit	$55.00	300
	Private Insurer HBAI code visit	$21.00	200
	Total Visits		2550
	85% of Visits Paid		$100,852.50
Variable 1	Contribution Margin/Net	150	(conservative offset or increase in year for Medical Provider: dual visit, optimal coding, group visit, increased access)
	Medical Provider Per Visit Reimbursement Average	$42.00	
		$6,300	$6,300
	BHP Level Net Revenue		**$107,153**
	Doctorate Level Net Revenue		$107,153
	Masters Net Revenue (usually pays between 10 and 20% less for private payers; 25% less for Medicare; these calculations based on 85% of physician fee schedule)	$107,153	$91,080
Variable 2	Grant funding	5,000	
	For small practices, grant funding may be essential for expansion and sustainability		
	Total Net Doctorate Level Revenue		**$112,153**
	Total Net Masters Level Revenue		**$96,080**
	Doctorate Level BHP (1.0 FTE)	$80,000.00	
	Benefits	$11,000.00	
	Total compensation	$91,000.00	

	Masters Level BHP (1.0 FTE)	$45,000.00	
	Benefits	$11,000.00	
	Total compensation	$56,000.00	
	Coding & billing expense	$5,046.86	
	Total Expenses Doctorate Level		$96,046.86
	Total Expenses Masters Level		$61,046.86
	Doctorate Level BHP Loss		**$16,106.00**
	Masters Level BHP Revenue		**$35,033**

*Revenue may be improved when independent practice sites consider the following:
Addition of another PCP
Addition of Grant Funding
Growth of Practice
Value/Cost of Benefits
Cost Benefits of Integrating Behavioral Health
Improvement of Provider and Staff Satisfaction
Improved Patient Outcomes
Professional and State Recognition for Integration and Health Home Development
Exapansion of Medical Visits, Group Visits, Medical Education, Community Outreach
Medicare Fee Schedule Reimbursement Percentage for Doctoral Level BHPs

We'd like to thank Dr. Glenn Kotz, MD and Dr. Corey D. Smith, PsyD, who provided information on their experiences and partnership in the development of integrated behavioral health at Mid Valley Family Practice in Basalt, Colorado.

Appendix 7H.
Return on Investment (ROI), Cost Savings, and Cost Offset

To take this business approach further, you may wish to calculate your return on investment in terms of earned income. Let's use a traditional example of integrated behavioral health (IBH) services to exemplify ROI.

Your behavioral health provider (BHP) treats 10 direct billable patients per day on average, with 2 dual-visit patients per day with the primary care provider (PCP) (both collaborate during the same appointment with the patient, working as a team for the presenting problem). At 5 billable patients coded as a 90832, you will receive approximately $311.35 and at 5 billable 96152, you will receive $105.25, equaling $416.60. The additional revenue from the dual PCP visits of $50.00 are due to upcoding and direct billable service. Thus, the BHP has $466.60 as monies earned for the day.

If we assume the BHP works 19 days in a month, then the monthly earnings will be $8,865.40. The BHP earns $65,000 per year with benefits and other nonsalary compensation of $25,000 for a total of $90,000. Thus, your fiscal cost per month is $7,500.

Return on Investment (ROI) Yearly Formula:

ROI: [$8,865.40 × 12 = $106,384.80] − $90,000
= $16,384.80

$$\frac{\text{gain from program} - \text{cost of program}}{\text{Cost of program}} = \frac{.182 \times 100}{\$90,000} = 18\% \text{ return}$$

Return on Investment (ROI) Monthly Formula:

ROI: $8,865.40 − $7,500

$$\frac{\text{gain from program} - \text{cost of program}}{\text{Cost of program}} = \frac{1,365}{7,500} = .182 \times 100 = 18\% \text{ return}$$

$7,500

With this calculation, the BHP is demonstrating an 18% fiscal return, which means for every $1 you spend in the program, the monthly return is an additional 18 cents. This equals an annual return of $16,200. Depending on earnings and fiscal costs of employees or programs, the ratio may not demonstrate earnings. In this scenario, the BHP may better demonstrate value through cost savings, cost offset, or a more well-developed pro forma (See Appendix 7G).

COST SAVINGS

In addition to direct revenue formulas, organizations may wish to calculate ROI through cost savings. Cost savings may be calculated through multiple analyses. Below is a generally accepted approach to calculating cost savings. Cost-savings calculations are important for all integrated care programs and payment models to view potential sustainability.

ROI Cost-Savings Formula:

$$\text{ROI:} \quad \frac{\text{cost savings attributed to program}}{\text{cost of program}}$$

This formula converts program impact into dollars. First, select a sample of patients for inclusion on the ROI analysis. This may be through a specific population health management project completed or from the patients, which were served by the BHP over a specific period of time (consult all your data sources including the electronic health record, practice management system, etc.).

Collect relevant data on these metrics: number of diagnoses, utilization of healthcare services, emergency department visits, PCP visits, diagnostic services, etc. Determine a comparison group to review data against as measurement. The comparison group may be the same group at a different period of time (prior to IBH intervention) or a similar patient sampling (similar data), which were not served by behavioral health. Then calculate the cost differential of the patients and divide by the cost of the program.

Now, let's take this same IBH provider above and view the ROI impact through the lens of the healthcare industry and a cost-savings initiative.

Prior to implementing IBH within the primary care office, Dr. Smith's panel was reviewed for potential cost-savings metrics. It was identified that Dr. Smith was seeing 200 duplicated patients per month who average 2.5 visits per month, equaling 500 encounters per month, and 100 unduplicated patients per month, with a total of 600 encounters per month.

This was a concern for Dr. Smith and his practice. Duplicated patients are typically indicative of complicated chronic conditions having high ongoing care needs and high costs to the healthcare industry. There may be deeper implications related to outcome management of these conditions, quality of life, and high utilization of health care services. Further, dependent on your billing, duplicated patients are not always billable per month and this also blocks other patients who need to access care. Instead, potential new patients and unduplicated patients reach out to Emergency Departments or urgent care clinics for their primary healthcare needs. In this example, you can also choose to complete an

ROI analysis to identify Dr. Smith's change in earned income through integrating behavioral health.

If we identify Dr. Smith's 200 duplicated patients per month as high utilizers and give them an average healthcare dollar cost of $85.00 per visit, these patients are costing the healthcare industry $42,500 per month/$510,000 per year (500 encounters x $85.00 = $42,500 per month x 12 = $510,000), focusing on Dr. Smith's encounters only.

After Dr. Smith brings on an IBH provider, the provider is able to see the 200 duplicated patients for health behavior change and chronic care management, using average billable visits of $45.00 per visit (due to use of mix of coding). The IBH provider sees 100 of the patients 2 times per month for 6 months and 100 patients 1 time per month. This transition of care cost $9,000 per month/$54,000 per year for half of the patients and $4,500 per month/$54,000 per year for the second half, totaling $13,500 per month/$108,000 per year.

Thus, the cost-savings equations are:

ROI Cost-Savings Yearly Formula:

ROI: $510,000 - $108,000 = $402,000

$$\frac{\text{cost savings attributed to program}}{\text{cost of program } \$90,000} = 4.4 \times 100 = 440\% \text{ cost savings on the initiative.}$$

ROI Cost-Savings Monthly Formula:

ROI: $42,500 - $13,500 = $29,000

$$\frac{\text{cost savings attributed to program}}{\text{cost of program } \$7,500} = 3.8 \times 100 = 380\% \text{ cost savings on the initiative.}$$

In other words, for every $1 spent on the IBH program, you save $4 in healthcare dollars. Thus, the cost savings is paying for the IBH service and then some.

Further, this assistance allowed Dr. Smith to see the patients who were not being seen, identify new patients, and provide more in-depth visits with patients he has been wanting to help manage more closely. Dr. Smith's new unduplicated visits moved to 300 at an average rate of $85.00 per visit. Overall, this demonstrated a return on investment for Dr. Smith, increased access to care, and provided a reduction in health care costs for the industry.

ROI: COST OFFSET

In IBH programs, medical cost offset may be a valuable asset to highlight, especially if you are working with health plans or medical homes following the Triple Aim. A general definition of cost offset is *the offset of decreased medical utilization based on the intervention*. An integrated care total offset occurs when general healthcare savings are identified as exceeding the cost of the integrated care intervention. This offset effectively results in paying for the intervention. It is important to recognize that cost savings does not always equal full cost offset.

For IBH programs attached to insurance companies, Accountable Care Organizations, Federally Qualified Health Centers, and other large healthcare entities with data sharing, the cost offset calculations may be best if they utilize the estimate of the intervention, health metric data, and quality adjusted life years (QALY).

To estimate a cost of an intervention, programs identify fixed time start-up costs, annual costs, and per patient variable costs. Then, to approximate the offset post intervention implementation, programs collect healthcare expenditure data from each patient inclusive of emergency room visits, pharmaceuticals, primary and specialty care visits, etc. Often costs may be calculated by what is shared and borne by a health plan entity. In addition, many will use QALY which is a measure of disease burden for both quality and quantity of life lived to assist in identifying the value of an intervention, cost-effectiveness, for the healthcare industry.

CHAPTER 8
Measuring Your Program's Impact

> **BOTTOM LINE, UP FRONT**
> - Calculating various returns on investment (ROIs) (direct and indirect revenue, cost savings, cost offset), developing pro formas, and evaluating your clinical outcomes are needed to assess your program.
> - Use a Triple or Quadruple Aim approach.
> - Ensure you have dedicated personnel and processes to conduct program evaluation.
> - Evaluate all metrics: implementation, process, operational, and outcome metrics.

It is important to measure the effectiveness of your program initially and continuously so you can improve it over time. Chapters 6 and 7 provide several basic methods and tools for measuring the IBH program's performance. We believe calculating various ROIs (direct and indirect revenue, cost savings, cost offset), developing pro formas, and evaluating your clinical outcomes are necessary minimum benchmarks for program assessment.

Several other program assessment methods have been discussed in the literature that we will briefly review in this chapter. These include CJ Peek's 3-world model (clinical, operational, financial perspectives) and the Triple Aim model (improved patient care experience, improved health of populations, decreased cost of care; See Tables 8.1 and 8.2).[1,2,3] Note that some have recently added a Fourth Aim—calling it the "Quadruple Aim"—which includes physician satisfaction, making the point that unhappy, burned-out physicians are a threat to the other three aims, not to mention a danger to the occupational health of physicians themselves.[4]

Make it a priority to have relevant stakeholders agree on a plan for collecting outcome metrics before starting your program. Some of these data may already be captured by your electronic health record (EHR) or financial accounting systems. Some of the clinical data (outcome metrics) you might want to collect probably are not being collected. For example, routine screening data can be collected by a practice's front desk or medical assistant staff, but these tasks need to be fully integrated into the workflow of clinical operations and into specific employees' tasks in order to be successfully adopted as a standard part of your practice. A well-developed EHR helps this process immensely. Therefore, review your strategy for collecting and reporting outcome metrics is shared with staff members, as they can provide feedback about how this information would be most helpful for their quality improvement efforts.

Clinical outcome metrics PCPs use (e.g., PHQ-9 or GAD-7 change score, Body Mass Index [BMI]) must be easily collected/scored, and relevant for quality improvement (i.e., formatted to inform PCPs about their patients' response to treatment).

There also are other standard (and free) measures of progress that you may elect to use when launching IBH. Changes in general health conditions probably will continue being assessed by your PCPs (e.g., biometrics like blood pressure, body mass index, and Hemoglobin A1c), and as we have described, the BHP may assist in delivering nonpharmacological treatments for these conditions, which may be captured by changes in biometrics. However, IBH may also deliver other clinical outcomes of interest. For example, consider measuring patients' quality of life (e.g., the 12-Item Short-Form Health Survey, SF-12[2]) or use standard measurement tools that are more specific to the general health condition (e.g., for chronic pain, consider using the PEG: A Three-Item Scale Assessing Pain Intensity and Interference[3]).

In addition to determining the metrics you want to collect, it is important to have someone dedicated to the quality assurance and analysis of those metrics. This data analyst works with managers or program directors to aggregate, analyze, and report metrics in a way that clinical and business staff can draw useful conclusions and plan changes. This might be your finance, quality improvement, or management staff, who will likely need some input and guidance on arranging and analyzing medical data. (See Chapter 5 for policy and other administrative and assessment responsibilities of this staff member). The methods by which smaller medical homes monitor their IBH program may differ substantially from larger organizations' methods. However, a few commonalities apply to all practices. Monitoring metrics can be done by case-sampling approaches (randomly selecting 100 cases and reviewing them based on the factors below), or more comprehensive data analysis approaches similar to those discussed in Chapters 6 and 7. Consider the following overarching framework that follows the Triple (and Quadruple) Aim:

1. Select implementation and process metrics, then focus on operational and performance metrics that help you understand your outcomes.
2. Calculate healthcare quality metrics.
3. Calculate staff and patient satisfaction metrics.
4. Calculate financial and resource costs versus gains.

IMPLEMENTATION METRICS AND PROCESS METRICS

Implementation metrics help you gauge your readiness to collect all other metrics. Implementation metrics may include determining whether:
- Leadership supports the IBH program and someone has oversight of product line;
- The right IBH provider has been selected and trained to meet product line goals;
- Funding for the IBH program is secured or there is a process in place for IBH service billing;
- Materials/equipment/space are available to seamlessly accommodate the IBH service; and
- Administrative policies, standard operating procedures, and business rules are in place that are clear regarding who is to do what and when for the IBH service.

Process metrics help you determine if your IBH product line:
- Maintains high fidelity to the core components of the service delivery model; and
- Is reaching the intended population (e.g., everyone with depression and diabetes).

You might consider using the National Committee for Quality Assurance (NCQA) 2014 criteria for behavioral health services as listed in Table 11.1 as a guide for devising additional IBH process metrics. Such metrics would keep you informed as to whether you are maintaining an IBH product line that continuously supports your medical home model.

OPERATIONAL METRICS AND OUTCOME METRICS

Operational metrics inform you about outcome metrics or the bottom line results that are of interest to patients, healthcare staff, administrators, and payers. These metrics may include:
- Numbers and types of referrals made to IBH;
- Numbers and types of referrals IBH has been unable to effect;
- Number and types of inappropriate referrals to IBH;
- Appointment wait length;
- Number of patients seen (i.e., productivity);
- Average number of visits/patient;
- Number of patients treated with meds; and
- Number of patients referred for outside services.

There are obviously many outcome variables that one can measure. Broad categories of outcome metrics include:
- Clinical outcomes: Improvement as assessed by objective measures for both mental (e.g., PHQ9s, GAD7s, functional status) and general health conditions

TABLE 8.1. Process and Operational Metrics within the Triple Aim Approach

Triple Aim Goal	Metric
Experience of Care	• Percent of patients asked to sign a release of information consent to allow agencies to exchange information • Percent of patients who sign a release of information consent • Frequency of contacting patients' other providers to coordinate care • Referral "hit rate"—the number of PCP-referred patients who actually accept the referral or warm handoff • Percent of patients who were asked to complete a healthcare satisfaction measure • Percent of patients who completed a healthcare satisfaction measure • Reasons patients did not complete satisfaction measure • Amount of time (e.g., same day, 3 days out) to next available IBH appointment • Patient educational materials are culturally appropriate and written in a language and at a level that best meets the patients' needs • Availability of staff who speak the same language as the population being served
Population Health	• Number of patients seen by the BHP in a week/month/quarter • Percent of patients seen in IBH who were screened for a given problem (e.g., depression) • Percent of patients who screen positive for a problem • Percent of patients who screened positive who were referred to the BHP for further assessment or intervention • Reason patients who screen positive were not referred to BHP for further assessment or intervention • Average number of clinic visits per patient per quarter (are those who need to be seen to ensure ongoing good health coming?) • Reasons patients with a given problem (e.g., diabetes) are not attending clinic appointments per recommended guidelines • Percent of PCP patients who have been referred for IBH (IBH service penetration rate) • Percent of PCP patients who have been treated by BHP • Percent of PCP patients—by diagnosis or panel—who *should have* been referred for IBH (are patients receiving appropriate evidence-based care?) • Percent of patients with a clearly documented integrated treatment plan
Cost	• Percent of patients who were referred to the BHP who kept the appointment (patients with poor follow-up may have worse health, therefore demanding a higher overall treatment cost from the payer) • Percent of patients who kept initial BHP appointment that were seen more than once • Percent of patients who were referred for a BH appointment outside of the primary care clinic • Percent of patients who were referred that kept the BH appointment outside of the primary care clinic • Type and duration of IBH treatment • Percent of patients newly prescribed psychotropic medication • Is psychotropic medication prescription being filled by the patient? • Number and type of diagnosis for patients who have high emergency room utilization • Number and type of diagnosis for patients who have higher hospital readmissions

and health behaviors (e.g., Hemoglobin A1c, cholesterol levels, smoking status, alcohol use, blood pressure, weight). See Table 8.3.
- Financial outcomes: Programmatic financial performance, average revenue/cost per patient, overhead costs, etc. See ROI Section of Chapter 7 and Appendices 7G and 7H.
- Health services outcomes: Change in frequency of medical visits, changes in ER visits/hospitalizations, total cost of care per unit time per patient, etc. See Section III.
- Clinician and staff job satisfaction/burnout: Consider the Burnout Inventory[5] and other scales that are fairly straightforward and standardized, and that help the leaders of the healthcare organization understand how they can improve operations and delivery of services.

Tables 8.1 and 8.2 present many possible process, operational, and outcome metrics a practice may choose to track given the unique goals of their IBH and medical home services.

TABLE 8.2. Outcome Metrics within the Triple Aim Approach

Triple Aim Goal	Metric
Experience of Care	- Level of patient satisfaction with access to general health services - Level of patient satisfaction with accessibility to IBH services - Level of patient satisfaction with effectiveness of physical health services - Level of patient satisfaction with effectiveness of IBH services - Level of PCP satisfaction with delivery of IBH services - Level of medical home staff knowledge and comfort level in IBH service provision
Population Health	- Patient quality of life functioning (e.g., score on a quality of life measure) - Patient mental health functioning (e.g., score on a mental health measure) - Patient general health status - Patient general health indicators (e.g., body mass index, waist girth, weight, blood pressure, blood glucose levels, lipid levels, pain level, alcohol use, physical activity, tobacco use) - Percent of improvement of number of enrollees in a given measure (e.g., body mass index or tobacco use) compared to previous year
Cost	- Annual percent increase in per-capita costs - Emergency room visits per 100 enrollees per year for any reason - Emergency room visits per 100 enrollees per year for mental health presentation alone - Frequency of psychiatric hospital admissions - Frequency of hospital admissions - Number and severity of general health and BH relapses - Rate of appropriate psychotropic prescription - Decreased overall specialty healthcare use

TABLE 8.3. Quality Metrics Resources

Electronic Health Record (EHR) Incentive Programs Patient Protection and Affordable Care Act (PPACA) Stage 2	• www.cms.gov/Regulations-and-Guidance/Legislation/ EHRIncentivePrograms/Recommended_Core_Set.html • www.cms.gov/Regulations-and-Guidance/Legislation/ EHRIncentivePrograms/eCQM_Library.html • www.cms.gov/Regulations-and-Guidance/Legislation/ EHRIncentivePrograms/CMS_EHR_Listserv.html • www.samhsa.gov/data/meaningful-use • www.cms.gov/Regulations-and-Guidance/Legislation/ EHRIncentivePrograms/index.html?redirect=/ ehrincentiveprograms • www.healthit.gov/
Preventive Care and Screening	• www.healthcare.gov/preventive-care-benefits/ • www.hhs.gov/healthcare/facts/timeline/index.html • www.hhs.gov/healthcare/facts/factsheets/2010/07/ preventive-services-list.html
CMS Clinical Quality Metrics	• www.cms.gov/Regulations-and-Guidance/Legislation/ EHRIncentivePrograms/ClinicalQualityMeasures.html • www.cms.gov/Regulations-and-Guidance/Legislation/ EHRIncentivePrograms/ReportingCQMsin2015.html • www.cms.gov/Medicare/Medicare-Fee-for-Service-Payment/sharedsavingsprogram/Quality_Measures_ Standards.html
Healthcare Effectiveness Data and Information Set (HEDIS)	• www.ncqa.org/HEDISQualityMeasurement/ HEDISMeasures/HEDIS2016.aspx
Patient-Centered Medical Home (PCMH)	• www.ncqa.org/Programs/Recognition/Practices/ PatientCenteredMedicalHomePCMH.aspx • https://pcmh.ahrq.gov • www.jointcommission.org/accreditation/primary_care_ medical_home_certification_option_for_hospitals.aspx
HRSA Clinical and Financial Performance Measures Uniform Data System (UDS)	• http://bphc.hrsa.gov/qualityimprovement/ performancemeasures/index.html • http://bphc.hrsa.gov/datareporting/reporting/index.html
Consumer Assessment of Healthcare Providers and Systems (CAHPS)	• http://acocahps.cms.gov/Content/Default.aspx
Accountable Care Organization (ACO) Shared Savings	• www.cms.gov/Medicare/Medicare-Fee-for-Service-Payment/sharedsavingsprogram/Quality-Measures-Standards.html
Joint Commission (JCAHO)	• www.jointcommission.org/performance_measurement. aspx
Agency for Healthcare Research and Quality (AHRQ)	• http://integrationacademy.ahrq.gov/atlas • http://integrationacademy.ahrq.gov/atlas/frameworkIBHC
Physician Quality Reporting System (PQRS)	• www.cms.gov/Medicare/Quality-Initiatives-Patient-Assessment-Instruments/PQRS/index.html

(Continued on next page)

National Quality Strategy	• www.ahrq.gov/workingforquality/ • www.cms.gov/Medicare/Quality-Initiatives-Patient-Assessment-Instruments/QualityInitiativesGenInfo/CMS-Quality-Strategy.html • www.samhsa.gov/data/national-quality-strategy • www.samhsa.gov/data/national-quality-forum-nqf
Substance Abuse and Mental Health Services Administration (SAMHSA) National Behavioral Health Quality Framework and Data Information	• www.samhsa.gov/data/national-quality-strategy • www.samhsa.gov/data/national-behavioral-health-quality-framework • www.samhsa.gov/data/node/20

Table 8.3 includes several additional resources related to measuring quality. Consider reviewing these resources as you devise your program measurement plan. See Chapters 6 and 7 for additional information on using data and metrics to improve your IBH program. Additional information on metrics can be found in the Partners in Health Interagency Toolkit at http://calmhsa.org/wp-content/uploads/2013/04/IBHP_Interagency_Collaboration_Tool_Kit_2013.pdf.

OTHER TOOLS FOR PROGRAM EVALUATION

In this section, we included a few additional tools, as many business professionals we know prefer to use tools like these for any new initiative, pet project, pilot, or process improvement project.

There are many other ways to evaluate your program, including the extent to which the IBH program is integrated and the fidelity of your BHP's practice skills (for the PCBH model). Many clinics have found practice assessments and toolkits helpful in their first steps for developing integration. Consider reviewing SAMHSA, IHI, and AHRQ for various practice assessments. These practice assessments may highlight site-specific areas for recognizing where you are in relationship to integration, areas to target change for integration efforts, and ways to monitor development. For example, the Practice Improvement Profile (PIP) is a 10-minute, six domain, 30-item web-based measure of level of integration based on the key clauses from C.J. Peek's Lexicon of Collaborative Care (2013): www.uvm.edu/~pip/pip.php.

The Primary Care Behavioral Health Provider Adherence Questionnaire (PPAQ) is a 48-item measure of the BHP's fidelity to the PCBH model. It takes less than 20 minutes to complete and is available here: http://integrationacademy.ahrq.gov/content/Assessing%20Provider%20Adherence%20to%20Integrated%20Care%20Development%20of%20the%20Primary%20Care%20Behavioral.

One framework for assessing programs was published as "RE-AIM." This analytic approach includes reach, effectiveness, adoption, implementation, and maintenance aspects of program operations.[6,7] It has been validated and used widely to evaluate the delivery of clinical services and to understand the impact of various factors on program implementation.[8] Another commonly used approach to ongoing program refinement is the Plan-Do-Study-Act (PDSA) cycle.[9] This is a low-tech process that office staff and managers can learn quickly and effectively use to evaluate a specific process, like screening for depression, and collect focused data, uncover glitches, and improve processes at whatever points need optimization. We add these two models knowing that one approach to program measurement does not suit all medical homes.

References

1. Peek, CJ, Heinrich, RL. Building a collaborative healthcare organization: From idea to invention to innovation. *Family Systems Medicine*. 1995;13(3-4):327-342. DOI: 10.1037/h0089218.
2. Peek, CJ. Planning care in the clinical, operational, and financial worlds. In Kessler R. and Stafford D. eds. *Collaborative Medicine Case Studies: Evidence in Practice*. New York: Springer;2008:25-26.
3. Berwick DM, Nolan TW, Whittington J. The triple aim: care, health, and cost. *Health Aff*. 2008;27(3):759-769. DOI: 10.1377/hlthaff.27.3.759.
4. Bodenheimer T, Sinsky C. From triple to quadruple aim: care of the patient requires care of the provider. *Ann Fam Med*. 2014;12(6):573-576. DOI: 10.1370/afm.1713.
5. Maslach, C, Jackson SE, Leiter MP. Maslach Burnout Inventory. (3rd ed.). Palo Alto, CA: Consulting Psychologists Press; 1996.
6. Glasgow RE, McKay HG, Piette JD, Reynolds KD. The RE-AIM framework for evaluating interventions: what can it tell us about approaches to chronic illness management? *Patient Educ Couns*. 2001;44(2):119-127.
7. Kessler RS, Purcell EP, Glasgow RE, Klesges LM, et al. What does it mean to "employ" the RE-AIM model? *Eval Health Prof*. 2013;36(1):44-66. DOI: 10.1177/0163278712446066.
8. Kirchner JE, Ritchie MJ, Pitcock JA, Parker LE, et al. Outcomes of a partnered facilitation strategy to implement primary care-mental health. *J Gen Intern Med*. 2014; 29 Suppl 4:904-912 DOI: 10.1007/s11606-014-3027-2.
9. Taylor MJ, McNicholas C, Nicolay C, Darzi A, et al. Systematic review of the application of the plan-do-study-act method to improve quality in healthcare. *BMJ Qual Saf*. 2014;23(4): 290-98. DOI: 10.1136/bmjqs-2013-001862.

CHAPTER 9
Hiring

> **BOTTOM LINE, UP FRONT**
> - Choose personnel who will thrive in patient-centered, team-oriented clinical settings marked by rapid-paced operations, unpredictability, and variety.
>
> - Prerequisite skills and experience in integrated care are paramount, along with the "right" personality attributes. Use a lock-and-key model; the behavioral health provider (BHP) needs to be a good fit for this work.
>
> - At all costs, try not to hire any BHP without having the individual observe another BHP who conducts the same model—even if that observation occurs in another healthcare system (public or private) or involves reviewing online videos of the model you select.

In our experience, you should expect some degree of turnover among the BHP and the medical home staff as you implement integrated care.[1] In some organizations, we have observed up to a 30% turnover rate for BHPs hired to conduct the primary care behavioral health (PCBH) model. As advised by the Institute for Healthcare Improvement (IHI), if medical home staff members do not adapt to your organizational initiatives (i.e., providing integrated care), it is advisable to let them go and hire new professionals who are willing to advance these objectives.[1] Ultimately, medical home staff (including BHPs) who lack full commitment to implement these new models of care may conceal it, or outwardly oppose your initiatives. All of these employee behaviors may bear negative effects on customer service, patient care, and relations within and outside your organization.

GET THE RIGHT PEOPLE ON THE BUS

In the U.S. military, a common phrase heard around leadership planning tables is, "If you get the right people on the bus, everything else falls into place." Once those people are on the bus, you also have to ensure they are placed in the "right" seats. A few straightforward business actions described in this chapter and the next, such as personnel selection, training, and management, will help you accomplish this. Unfortunately we are aware of no reliable empirical study that details how to select the best personnel for behavioral health service delivery in primary care. However, experts have made several recommendations over the past two decades that align with our experiences of delivering and training others to deliver evidence-based behavioral health services in primary care.[2,3,4]

> *Unfortunately we are aware of no reliable empirical study that details how to select the best personnel for behavioral health service delivery in primary care.*

WHO ARE THE "RIGHT" PEOPLE?

1. Scout for employees who are hard-working, responsible, flexible, and forward-thinking.
2. Find people who clearly work well in teams—who are confident and likable.
3. Hire employees who genuinely care about what they do. These professionals and paraprofessionals already operate with these positive work habits because these habits are consistent with their personal values.
4. Keep in mind that conscientiousness is the personality trait most closely and consistently associated with high job performance.
5. You want people in your medical home who have an internal compass consistent with medical home concepts.
6. Hire BHPs who have sufficient training and the *right* personality characteristics for this work. If some of the skills are lacking, that's fine, you can tap into available training resources (See Chapter 10).

> *You want people in your medical home who have an internal compass consistent with medical home concepts.*

By hiring people who already demonstrate the positive characteristics listed on the next page, you ensure your organization's training teams and programs have time and resources to address higher-level problems instead of spending time on basic or remedial issues. Hiring the "right" people means resources can be devoted to the initiatives the company values, and less time is wasted grappling with personnel issues.

Robinson and Reiter[4] developed a helpful list of candidate interview questions. (See Appendix 9A). This list also includes examples of answers you want from candidates, indicating they are likely to be good hires, and answers you

The Right Stuff

The most successful mental health professionals to recruit for medical homes are:
- ☐ Flexible;
- ☐ Adaptive;
- ☐ Interested in learning and teaching;
- ☐ Sociable;
- ☐ Personable;
- ☐ Adept at thinking quickly, particularly without preparation;
- ☐ Conscientious;
- ☐ Able to multitask;
- ☐ Able to handle stress, chaos, and unpredictability calmly and effectively;
- ☐ Confident, but balanced with some humility;
- ☐ Genuine;
- ☐ Empathic;
- ☐ Comfortable in fast-paced environments;
- ☐ Values the mind/body connection;
- ☐ Non-judgmental;
- ☐ Extroverted; and
- ☐ Not intimidated by working with other specialties.

Seek potential mental health providers who have sufficient prerequisite skills:
- ☐ Builds and maintains positive relationships, particularly in ambiguous or uncertain situations;
- ☐ Ability to accurately communicate complex concepts in very few words;
- ☐ Learns quickly;
- ☐ Possesses medical knowledge;
- ☐ Strong diagnostic skills;
- ☐ Strong assessment skills;
- ☐ Strong knowledge and skill in implementing brief behavioral and cognitive interventions;
- ☐ Strong motivational interviewing skills;
- ☐ Solid understanding of the medical model (e.g., assess, treat, monitor, repeat);
- ☐ Adroit at teaching patients and medical team members; and
- ☐ Consultation experience.

> **Red Flags**
>
> If possible, avoid hiring staff with these personality red flags:
> - ☐ Rigidity;
> - ☐ Overconfidence;
> - ☐ Insistence on being right;
> - ☐ Self-aggrandizing;
> - ☐ Needing excessive preparation or time to perform optimally;
> - ☐ Non-adaptive; and
> - ☐ Easily or often defensive.
>
> Select mental health professionals who possess sufficient training prerequisites (See Table 2.1). Avoid people who:
> - ☐ Shy away from being observed and co-treating with PCPs;
> - ☐ Love delivering psychotherapy;
> - ☐ Convey the need to "own" their own caseload of patients;
> - ☐ Are sensitive to power and authority;
> - ☐ Assume too much responsibility for their patients;
> - ☐ Foster excessive patient dependency on himself/herself;
> - ☐ Does not take feedback well;
> - ☐ Lack experience and desire to work in teams;
> - ☐ Lack experience in behavioral medicine; and
> - ☐ Are unable to analyze and conceptualize patients' biopsychosocial factors.

don't want, suggesting you might pass on that individual. Consider using these questions and developing similar tools based on the skills and personnel characteristics listed above. We also have included additional questions that we have used in the field (Appendix 9B), and two sample job descriptions for hiring the BHP (Appendices 9C–9D).

Shifting to a medical home model of primary care and introducing IBH triggers a shift in healthcare culture on multiple levels. Culture clash between primary care and mental health has been identified as a common barrier to successful integration.[1] To minimize this, hire people with prior experience in IBH. If you cannot find someone with prior experience, a second strategy may be to search for someone who has worked in multidisciplinary care settings. This may be behavioral health or other medical personnel who have experience working in the Emergency Department, in crisis units, in hospitals, or in other places that have team-based care. Often this is not possible, so consider hiring someone who meets the aforementioned personality characteristics criteria and a *stated desire* to work in a team-based primary care or medical setting. Regardless, we suggest providing subsequent training after hiring the BHP. We will discuss this more in the next chapter.

As a part of the hiring process, arrange for the potential BHP to shadow and observe someone working in the model you intend to launch. If you are starting a new program and have no other BHP for the prospective hire to observe, consider reviewing online videos of the respective model of care with your prospective hire. Several resources depict role-plays that are useful for hiring and training purposes. For the primary care behavioral health (PCBH) model of service delivery, consider viewing the following YouTube channels: NCR Behavioral Health and Primary Care Shrink. View the demos with applicants and ask them to discuss how the video reflects or does not reflect their prior experience and practice skills, and if they believe they can learn and appreciate this modality.

For the Care Management Model, have the prospective hires review a few research reports with you (e.g., "The Collaborative Care Model: An Approach for Integrating Physical and Mental Health Care in Medicaid Health Homes" [www.medicaid.gov/State-Resource-Center/Medicaid-State-Technical-Assistance/Health-Homes-Technical-Assistance/Downloads/HH-IRC-Collaborative-5-13.pdf] or *Respect-Mil: Primary Care Clinician's Manual* [www.pdhealth.mil/respect-mil/downloads/pcc_final.pdf]), then ask them how they would fit if hired to implement these protocols and serve in this role. See Chapter 10 for more on training resources and Chapter 11 to learn more about the process of helping your clinic staff acclimate to integrated care, as written from a PCP's perspective.

A few final words about interviewing. The more behavioral your interview is with the BHP candidate, the more accurate a conclusion you will make about their goodness-of-fit for your IBH program. As a part of the interview you might ask fund-of-knowledge questions about medical problems (e.g., What is hemoglobin A1C and why is it important in diabetes care? What are the common side effects of selective serotonin re-uptake inhibitors? Describe the underlying etiology that explains why patients experience difficulties with sleep onset and sleep maintenance in insomnia). While the BHP candidate can learn this kind of information if necessary (unlike the personal and professional characteristics we listed earlier), it is helpful if your applicant already possesses this knowledge.

It may also be helpful to use behavioral interview tasks such as:
- Providing the applicant with case vignettes and asking him or her to assign a diagnosis and brief treatment goals on the spot;
- Discussing a biopsychosocial case conceptualization for the vignette;

- Demonstrating how to give the PCP feedback about the case described in the vignette; and
- Discussing how he or she would help the patient learn about a particular mental health or general health condition.

It may be helpful to include someone with behavioral medicine knowledge (a PCP and another BHP experienced in IBH) while conducting the interview. It also may require the use of role play exercises to ascertain the information about the applicant that you need for making solid hiring decisions. Your selectiveness will pay off, trust us. If the applicant cannot do these tasks in the interview there is little chance he/she will be able to do them in "real-time."

LABOR TYPES AND COSTS

Regarding staffing ratios and caseload sizes, pair your BHP with specific PCPs and their medical home teams to ensure they work collaboratively. If your practice has a patient size of at least 3,000 patients, it can likely support 1.0 full-time employee (FTE) for the PCBH model or 1.0 FTE nurse plus an added 0.1 FTE psychiatrist who may work outside your practice (Care Management Model). If your medical home empanels 7,500+ patients, you may benefit from 2.0 FTEs—one from each of these models. Although standard staffing guidelines for medical family therapy (MedFT) have not been established, consider following these staffing ratios for MedFT as well. While all of these are general recommendations, also follow your business case analysis and business plan. If you choose a Care Management Model, consider hiring one nurse per 150–300 patients on psychotropic medications.

Beware of diminishing returns. To our knowledge, there are no known studies calculating cost and gain of specific staffing ratios, but studies have shown that even in clinics staffed with high numbers of BHPs, the IBH service may be underutilized.[5] In our experience, hiring fewer staff is safer until the BHPs are productive and well-utilized by your PCPs. This helps you rapidly intervene when you see something undesirable in your IBH service. Additionally, this pilot-style start enables you to avoid scaling the program before you have matured it.

What type of provider will be necessary to meet the needs and provide the services? It depends entirely on the type of model you launch (recall Figure 6.1). Cost still will be a factor. The Bureau of Labor Statistics provides a nationwide look at compensation levels by job title, but recognize that the local market will be the determining factor in your plan. Also consider that the job market for these innovative BHP positions is not well-published, standardized, or specified by the Bureau of Labor Statistics. Consider contacting any of the systems listed in Section III of this book to help develop salary ranges. The Department of Defense salary ranges are publically available. For PCBH programs, the salaries range from

$80,000 to $120,000 for 1.0 FTE depending on if you've hired a master's level or doctoral-level BHP. As you may have concluded by now, doctoral-level BHPs may cost you more in salary expenses. But, consider that the reasons for hiring a doctoral-level BHP versus a master's level mirror those which motivate practices to hire PCPs at a higher level (i.e., physician versus physician's assistant or nurse practitioner). There are costs and benefits to hiring BHPs at various levels. We advise you to think through these costs and benefits thoroughly, especially in light of the complexity of your patients, your program goals, and your payers (e.g., Medicare). For the nurses, these range from $60,000 to $90,000, depending on whether you've hired an LPN or RN.

We acknowledge that these salaries may be higher than some employers in the private sector will pay these professionals; locality is also a variable to consider. However, also consider that paying slightly higher salaries for these BHPs may be reasonable, as you are asking them to work to the peak of their credentials, to collaborate with other professionals through team workflow models, and to

TABLE 9.1. Training Needs and Credentials of Behavioral Health Providers (BHPs)

Role	Acceptable	Preferred	Precautions
Behavioral Health Consultant (PCBH)[2-4, 14-17]	Bachelor's degree or higher in nursing (in Canada); Master's degree or higher in professional or mental health counseling, or clinical social work; doctorate level behavioral health, clinical or counseling psychology AND License in one of these	Doctoral-level clinical psychologist with training, board certification and/or experience in health psychology or primary care psychology	This takes very specific training above and beyond the academic curricula of the LPN, BSN, MSW, PhD, PsyD programs; require that these hires have had some exposure to PCBH in graduate training; also require additional training for all hires for this model.
Co-located Specialty Mental Health[2]	Master's degree or higher in professional or mental health counseling, clinical social work or marriage and family therapy; doctoral-level clinical or counseling psychology, social work or psychiatry AND License in one of these	Psychologist or psychiatrist	The therapist *must* use evidence-based psychotherapy (preferably cognitive-behavioral therapy or behavioral therapy). A psychiatrist may provide consultation services to the PCPs in addition to seeing a full caseload of patients for therapy and/or medication management.

(Continued on next page)

TABLE 9.1. Training Needs and Credentials of BHPs (continued from previous page)

Role	Acceptable	Preferred	Precautions
Medical Family Therapist[11-13]	Master's degree or higher in professional or mental health counseling, clinical social work, counseling or clinical psychology, or marriage and family therapy AND License in one of these	Masters degree in marriage and family therapy with marriage; doctoral degree in clinical or counseling psychology specializing in marriage and family therapy	This takes very specific training above and beyond the academic curricula of the MSW, PhD, PsyD; and Masters in marriage and family therapy. All hires must have already completed a Medical Family Therapy (MedFT) Master's degree.
Care Manager[2, 6-10, 19, 20]	Certified medical assistant or higher medical or nursing credentials	LPN or RN	This is a narrow scope within nursing; must have population health interest; mental health background is *not* needed. Additional training about psychotropic medications and routinely using standardized outcome measures is needed.
Consulting Psychiatric Prescriber[2, 6-10, 18-20]	Psychiatric nurse practitioner; prescribing psychologist; psychiatrist	Psychiatrist	This service may be employed with or without a Care Facilitator and Care Management model
Reverse Integration/ Bidirectional Integration	Nurse Practitioner, Medical or Osteopathic Doctor AND License in one of these	Family Physician	Familiarity with psychotropic medications is very important as all patients seen will most likely be taking these; ability to work in multidisciplinary teams with specialty mental health providers

operate in new ways, as part of integrated care teams. Again, conduct your business case analysis, consult with an IBH subject matter expert, and communicate with the network of other organizations that have launched these models successfully to determine the salary. Clearly, you want to hire the highest-quality professional at the most reasonable and feasible cost.

A professional degree and license (if applicable) in a pertinent mental health field are the minimum credentials needed. Table 9.1 lists the various professions and the authors' recommendations regarding preferred and acceptable credentials. All professionals listed under "acceptable" have the legal permission to do this work. All of the professionals listed under "preferred" have this *and* subsequent supervised training that closely matches the type of work needed to operate effectively in an IBH program in a medical home. Table 9.1 was constructed considering:

1. Minimum standards for practicing the specialty independently and/or obtaining reimbursement from third-party payers;
2. Consideration of how each of these professionals' academic training addresses primary care; and
3. Research reports and our collective experience working within the integrated primary care field domestically and abroad and seeing which specialties easily succeed in a medical home setting, assuming all personality characteristics and clinical skills are equal.

References

1. Institute for Healthcare Improvement. *IHI 90-Day R&D Project Final Summary Report: Integrating Behavioral Health and Primary Care*. Cambridge, MA: Institute for Healthcare Improvement; March 2014. Available at www.ihi.org.
2. Gatchel RJ, Oordt MS. *Clinical Health Psychology and Primary Care: Practical Advice and Clinical Guidance for Successful Collaboration*. Washington, DC: American Psychological Association; 2003.
3. Hunter, CL, Goodie JL, Oordt MS, Dobmeyer, AC. *Integrated Mental Health in Primary Care: Step-by-Step Guidance for Assessment and Intervention*. Washington, DC: American Psychological Association; 2009.
4. Robinson P, Reiter J. *Behavioral Consultation and Primary Care: A Guide to Integrating Services* (2nd ed.). Geneva, Switzerland: Springer International Publishing; 2015.
5. Scharf DM, Eberhart NK, Hackbarth NS, et al. *Evaluation of the SAMHSA Primary and Behavioral Health Care Integration (PBHCI) Grant Program: Final Report (Task 13)*. Santa Monica, CA: RAND Corporation; 2014. http://www.rand.org/pubs/research_reports/RR546.html. Accessed April 24, 2015.
6. Belsher BE, Curry J, McCutchan P, et al. Implementation of a collaborative care initiative for PTSD and depression in the Army primary care system. *Social Work in Mental Health*. 2014;12(5-6):500-22. DOI:10.1080/15332985.2014.897673.
7. Katon WJ, Von Korff M, Lin EHB, et al. The Pathways Study: A randomized trial of collaborative care in patients with diabetes and depression. *Arch Gen Psychiatry*. 2004; 61(10): 1042-1049. DOI: 10.1001/archpsyc.61.10.1042.
8. Dietrich AJ, Oxman TE, William JW, et al. Re-engineering systems for the treatment of depression in primary care: cluster randomised controlled trial. *BMJ*. 2004; 329(7466):602. DOI: 10.1136/bmj.38219.481250.55.
9. Williams M, Angstman K, Johnson I, Katzelnick D. Implementation of a care management model for depression at two primary care clinics. *J Ambul Care Manage*. 2011;34(2):163-173. DOI: 10.1097/JAC.0b013e31820f63cb.
10. Cape J, Whittington C, Bower P. What is the role of consultation–liaison psychiatry in the management of depression in primary care? A systematic review and meta-analysis. *Gen Hosp Psychiatry*. 2010;32(3):246-54. DOI: 10.1016/j.genhosppsych.2010.02.003.

11. McDaniel SH, Doherty WJ, Hepworth J. *Medical Family Therapy and Integrated Care.* 2nd ed. Washington, DC: American Psychological Association; 2014.
12. McDaniel SH, Belar CD, Schroeder C, Hargrove DS, et al. A training curriculum for professional psychologists in primary care. *Professional Psychology: Research and Practice.* 2002;33(1):65-72. DOI: 10.1037/07357028.33.1.65.
13. McDaniel, SH, LeRoux P. An overview of primary care family psychology. *J Clin Psychol Med Settings.* 2007;14(1):23-32. DOI: 10.1007/s10880-006-9050-7.
14. Bryan CJ, Corso ML, Corso KA, Morrow CE, et al. Severity of mental health impairment and trajectories of improvement in an integrated primary care clinic. *J Consult Clin Psychol.* 2012; 80(3):396-403. DOI: 10.1037/a0027726.
15. Corso KA, Bryan CJ, Corso ML, et al. Therapeutic alliance and treatment outcome in the primary care mental health model. *Fam Sys Health.* 2012;30(2):87-100. DOI: 10.1037/a0028632.
16. Corso KA, Kanzler KA, Morrow CE, Corso ML, Ray-Sannerud B, Bryan CJ. Therapeutic alliance and training level. Poster session for the annual meeting of the Society of Behavioral Medicine; April 2012; New Orleans, LA.
17. Strosahl K. The psychologist in primary healthcare. In: Kent AJ, Hensen M, ed. *A Psychologist's Proactive Guide to Managed Mental Healthcare.* Hillsdale, NJ: Erlbaum; 2000: 87-112.
18. Lambert D, Hartley D. Linking primary care and rural psychiatry: Where have we been and where are we going? *Psychiatr Serv.* 1998;49(7):965-967. DOI: 10.1176/ps.49.7.965.
19. Zeidler Schreiter EA, Pandhi N, Fondow MDM, et al. Consulting psychiatry within an integrated primary care model. *J Health Care Poor Underserved.* 2013;24(4):1522–1530. DOI: 10.1353/hpu.2013.0178.
20. Kates N, Crustolo AM, Farrar S, Nikolaou L. Integrating mental health services into primary care: Lessons learnt. *Families, Systems, & Health.* 2001;19(1):5-12. DOI: 10.1037/h0089457.

Appendix 9A.
Interview Questions (and Desired Answers) for BHC Position Applicants.

What are your thoughts on the current state of mental health care in general?

Look for someone who sees problems with the specialty model of care and wants to try something different, though they may only have a vague idea of what that might involve. Candidates who say they want to see more patients or extend services to a greater percentage of the population or point to the importance of improving access to care through same-day visits are on the right track. On the other hand, candidates who complain about not getting satisfactory reimbursement or about restrictions from managed care might not possess the vision that makes a successful BHC.

Describe your ideal work situation, including the room and area of a building where you would like to work.

MH providers are usually trained to maintain private and quiet offices, so don't be surprised to hear this as an answer. However, the ideal candidate will say she likes to be in the middle of the action and thinks that's the best way to become a part of a team.

What types of patients are you most eager to see?

Be skeptical of candidates inclined toward a narrow specialty practice and/or the pursuit of non-clinical activities regarding select groups of patients (e.g., research, administration). Also, avoid candidates who may avoid or refuse to treat certain problems. All providers have a comfort zone clinically, but those with the widest zone and a willingness to expand it will work best as a BHC.

If you only had 15 minutes to spend with a patient experiencing insomnia and marital problems, what would you do?

Most interviewees will express surprise and perhaps uncertainty when asked to describe a 15-minute intervention, but nonetheless some answers are better than others. Look for answers that stick to the problems at hand and that end up with a reasonably clear self-management plan. A favorable candidate may suggest screening for common causes of insomnia, such as problematic work schedules or poor sleep hygiene habits, and then developing an intervention that addresses factors that may be triggering the insomnia. The candidate may also suggest exploring marital problems as a potential catalyst to the patient's issues with sleep and suggest a future check-in with the patient via a brief follow-up. Simply suggesting a referral for outside counseling is an insufficient answer.

If you were asked to consult with a PCP about an 8 year-old child with attention and behavior problems at school, what would you do?

Many MH providers have led a fairly specialized existence, so those who have worked primarily with adults might express unease when asked about working with children. However, strong candidates will be open to working with new populations and problems, and have at least a basic idea of how to help. For example, the applicant may identify ways he can help the PCP (e.g., contacting the child's teachers, recommending brief standardized assessment tools, meeting with parents, etc.), demonstrate an awareness of diagnostic criteria for child behavior problems, and/or show some familiarity with behavior modification techniques. A good follow-up question could be to ask the applicant what he would say to a PCP about a child that possibly had Attention Deficit Hyperactivity Disorder, Combined Type. Look for a familiarity with basic behavior change techniques and that ideally demonstrate an awareness of the time limitations in PC. Simply suggesting a referral for counseling or more evaluation is, again, an insufficient answer.

If you were asked to consult with a PCP about an obese, adult patient with diabetes who is non-compliant with treatment, what would you do?

As with previous questions, many candidates will issue a disclaimer that obesity and diabetes have not been mainstays of their past work, yet they should show some basic familiarity with both and a willingness to engage with the patient. Ideal answers will mention approaches such as motivational interviewing or psychological acceptance of chronic disease, or may reference collaborative goal-setting approaches. Exploration of the patient's mood (e.g., to assess for depression) would also be a reasonable part of the plan. Detailed understanding of the medical aspects of obesity and diabetes should not be expected.

If the clinic manager came to you and asked you to be the lead for the clinic in developing a clinical pathway for chronic pain, what would you do?

Relatively few candidates will be familiar with the term "clinical pathway", which means that the one who is may be a strong candidate (though one who isn't might still be a good candidate). If unfamiliar with the concept, a candidate should at least express an interest in learning about it. An impressive answer would include the importance of focusing on quality of life and functioning (in addition to pain intensity) as an outcome, and/or an awareness of the potential pitfalls of narcotic analgesics. Applicants who express an interest in or knowledge of novel interventions such as group visits will also likely be keepers. At a minimum, candidates should recognize chronic pain as something they can help with and be willing to work on issues at the systems-level. Candidates who say they would not feel able to take on such a task should lose favor.

Describe a project you initiated and then developed. It could be large or small, recent or from your past, and could be a work, school or volunteer project.

This question can help identify the self-starters among the applicants. This is an especially important trait for the BHC who is hired to develop a new service, since that requires the ability to form a clear vision for the service, the ability to work with other to develop it, and the persistence to stick with the plan despite any number of obstacles. However, BHCs hired into an existing service also benefit from this trait. Often there is only one BHC on the PC team, or only a small number of BHCs spread across a large medical staff, either of which can feel isolating at times. To succeed in such a situation, one needs to have self-starter qualities. Thus, individuals who can readily list work, school, or volunteer project(s) they have initiated and developed throughout their adult life might be good candidates to consider; those who struggle to think of any examples might not be. (With kind permission from Springer Science+Business Media: *Recruiting and Training a Behavioral Health Consultant*, January 1, 2016; Author, Patricia J. Robinson and Jeffrey T. Reiter.)

Appendix 9B.
Additional Interview Questions for Consideration

- Describe the role of a BH provider in conjunction with a medical clinic.
- Tell me what you know about healthcare reform and the role of behavioral health within medical settings.
  - Define integrated behavioral health.
- Tell me about your knowledge of the primary care provision of care experience.
  - What are your assumptions about it?
- What motivates you about working in primary care?
  - Why is it important for BH to be integrated into primary care?
- Tell me how BH providers can be utilized outside of mental health.
- What would you do to further integrate mental/behavioral health with medical care for our patients?
- Describe ways you would demonstrate team building.
  - Describe some ways a BHP would demonstrate collaborative care.
- Tell me about your knowledge of population health.
  - Any ideas on medical or dual diagnosis population health programs to implement?
  - Dual medical visits or groups to implement?
- What type of support would you like/expect from onsite administration?
- What would you say are your predominate strengths as a clinician/professional/manager?
- What type of support and relationship would be ideal for you with regard to our medical patients?
  - With regard to working with our medical team and providers?
- Describe how you would handle a situation where interprofessional ethics and/or legal requirements are different.
- Describe your comfort with working in a collaborative team approach to care with shared records and access.
- Have you ever worked in an electronic health record before?
  - Do you have any concerns related?
  - Do you have any concerns about sharing a medical record with primary care?
- Describe your familiarity with brief (at 15-30 minutes), solution-focused, evidence-based interventions.
  - Give an example of using a 15-minute intervention/appointment.
- Are you comfortable with being interrupted while you are providing care?
  - How would you handle being interrupted?

- How would you expect to be measured regarding outcomes and effectiveness?
- Where do you see yourself professionally in 5 years?
  - What types of support would you like to see related to this?
- Tell me about the professional organizations you are a member of or strive to be active in?
- What trainings or conferences do you believe would be helpful for you to function your best as a member of the integrated care team here?

Appendix 9C.
Sample Job Description for Primary Care BHP

Job Title: Primary Care Behavioral Health Provider
Department: Medical
Reports To: Site Behavioral Health Director and Medical Director

SUMMARY:

As part of the primary care treatment team, the provider identifies, triages and manages primary care patients with medical and behavioral health problems. In addition, the provider will utilize skill training through psycho-education and patient education strategies to develop patient self-management, population health programs, and will develop specific behavioral change plans for patients using best practice and brief evidence based treatment interventions.

ESSENTIAL DUTIES AND RESPONSIBILITIES:

- Assists in program development for groups (e.g.: pain, diabetes, weight loss, stress, etc.).
- Assesses the clinical status of patients referred by the primary care provider.
- Assists in the detection of "at risk" patients and prevents further psychological or physical deterioration.
- Assists primary health care providers in recognizing and treating mental disorders and psychosocial problems.
- Uses brief assessment tools with patients to assist with identifying concerns, triaging, and outcome measurements.
- Consults with physician supervisor as necessary and refers cases to specialty, case management, and other behavioral health providers as appropriate.
- Works with primary care team to treat and manage patients with chronic emotional and/or physical health problems efficiently and effectively.
- Assists in preventing relapse or morbidity in conditions that tend to recur over time.
- Operates within the provider care teams (e.g.: pods, teamlets).
- Improves clinical outcomes with high prevalence medical and mental health conditions.
- Connects with new and established patients regarding integrated care model and care team information.
- Evaluates patient care plans with primary care team.

- Attends provider meetings monthly. Provides education/training to medical providers 2x/year.
- Provides a minimum of two community education events (e.g.: stress management, diabetes, etc.) per year.
- Assists with process improvement teams and best practice development related to integrated care.
- Completes education for staff on topics selected with site administrators and/or supervisor during staff meetings and established education events (e.g.: communication, teamwork, team building).
- Teaches patients, families, and staff care, prevention, and treatment enhancement techniques.
- Accurately records patient history, exam notes, medication history, on-going care, and referrals in medical record (according to established format and workflows). Updates medical record as required.
- Attends and participates in meetings, team huddles, provider meetings, and Quality Assurance activities as required.
- Serves as a member of site committees as requested.
- Responds to patient or co-worker complaints and works toward a positive resolution of any dispute.
- Identifies problems related to patient services and makes recommendations for improvement.
- Participates in evaluation of peers and support staff.
- Completes behavioral modification plans.
- Assist with de-escalation and crisis intervention of patients in clinic as needed.
- Completes formal outreach and training to other integrated care providers 1x/year.
- Sustains productivity expectations established by Director and Site Administrator.
- Sustains motivation in organizations mission.
- Adherence to attendance policy.
- Other duties and responsibilities as designated by supervisor.

QUALIFICATIONS:

- Ability to work as a member of a team in order to solicit input from other affected departments or individuals, communicate pertinent information to other team members, and support team decisions.
- Ability to communicate effectively and exercise sound and responsible judgment.
- Excellent interpersonal skills, written and verbal. Ability to establish constructive working relationships with all levels of management and employees in a staff of varied and diverse backgrounds.

- Strong flexibility and teamwork skills to adapt to interprofessional and high productivity environments.
- Ability to handle difficult or confrontational situations in a calm, consistent, and equitable manner.
- Ability to read, analyze, and interpret business periodicals, professional journals, technical procedures, and governmental regulations.
- Ability to effectively represent the clinic's interests in the community; maintaining effective working relationships among public, private and professional groups.

EDUCATION AND/OR EXPERIENCE:
- Doctorate in clinical or counseling psychology, counseling, psychology, or behavioral health (preferred).
- Masters degree in social work, psychology, marriage and family.
- Nursing degree.
- Minimum two-years field experience.
- Preferred experience working in primary care or medical teams.

CERTIFICATES, LICENSES, REGISTRATIONS:
- Preferred current and active state practice license
- Licensed: clinical psychologist, social worker, professional counselor, marriage and family therapist, nurse
- License eligible (see above)

Appendix 9D. Sample Job Description for Director of Behavioral Health

Job Title: Director of Behavioral Health (e.g.: Director of Integrated Care Services)
Department: Behavioral Health/Administration
Reports To: Associate Corporate Medical Director and Chief Operations Officer

SUMMARY:

The Behavioral Health Director is responsible for planning, prioritizing, and implementing behavioral health and integrated care services. They work to provide behavioral health and administrative direction to the Behavioral Health program and lead efforts to build the culture of integrated care across providers, patients, clinics, systems, and organizations (e.g.: interagency collaborations and relationships). The Director is responsible for developing effective and consistent protocols, procedures, and policies pertaining to the behavioral health functions and ensures quality improvement and assurance. Further responsibilities may be inclusive of supervision, training, orientation/on-boarding, human resources directorship duties, and clinical oversight to ensure highest quality of evidence based care.

ESSENTIAL DUTIES AND RESPONSIBILITIES:

- Works with clinical sites to ensure high quality behavioral health services
- Develops policies, procedures, workflows, and electronic health record processes for integrated care
- Provides supervision and direction to behavioral health and site administration
- Reviews quality metrics monthly for reporting and individual provider/clinic review
- Develops new programs for furthering integration efforts
- Develops relationships with collaborative agencies
- Serves as a public liaison for behavioral health related concerns
- Participates on county, state, and/or federal level taskforces and coalitions for behavioral health integration, contracts, and policies
- Works directly with quality improvement officer/department to ensure program and provider metrics are reviewed regularly, support medical health and organization mission, and are reflective of quality care
- Exercises authority in making employee appointments, dismissals, and any other behavioral health personnel changes in cooperation with the Associate Corporate Medical Director, Human Resources Directors, and applicable Site Medical Administrator.

- Participates in Quality Assurance meetings, soliciting recommendations from other staff about necessary and appropriate Quality Assurance activities and in-service training to improve the behavioral health services provided by the clinics and tied to federal metric healthcare standards (e.g.: HEDIS, UDS, NCQA)
- Develop and monitor pro formas and budgets related to program and personnel for fiscal control of department
- Develops, reviews, approves, and monitors Behavioral Health protocols, procedures and evidence based practices in consultation with Associate Corporate Medical Director and operations team.
- Periodically reviews charts of Behavioral Health to assess consistency with agency and payor protocols and procedures
- Orients and extensively reviews new staff to assure competency. Participates in on-going evaluation and peer reviews.
- Works with corporate grant writing team in developing, presenting and implementing Behavioral Health grants.
- Liaison with community behavioral health agencies in conjunction with other behavioral health staff
- Responds to and resolves concerns about Behavioral Health Consultant personnel and the Behavioral Health Program in accordance with established clinic policies and procedures
- Conducts regular site visits to remote clinics to ensure Behavioral Health Program integration, utilization, model fidelity, and provide support and consultation to providers for culture change to integrated care
- Models expected professional and ethical conduct
- Other duties and responsibilities as assigned

QUALIFICATIONS:

- Knowledge of health care delivery and administration, as well as legal and ethical issues related to health care and integrated care.
- Ability to work with a team approach to management. Ability to work as a member of a team in order to solicit input from other affected departments or individuals, communicate pertinent information to other team members, and support team decisions.
- Ability to be persuasive and diplomatic in encouraging teamwork and cooperation in the pursuit of excellence in service.
- Ability to communicate effectively and exercise sound and responsible judgment.
- Excellent interpersonal skills, written and verbal. Ability to establish constructive working relationships with all levels of management and employees in a staff of varied and diverse backgrounds.

- Ability to handle difficult or confrontational situations in a calm, consistent, and equitable manner.
- Ability to supervise others and delegate effectively.
- Ability to effectively present information and respond to questions from groups of managers, clients, customers, and the general public.
- Ability to read, analyze, and interpret business periodicals, professional journals, technical procedures, and governmental regulations.
- Ability to effectively represent the organization's interests in the community.
- Ability to maintain effective working relationships among public, private, and professional groups.

EDUCATION and/or EXPERIENCE:
- A minimum of 5 years experience supervising personnel
- A minimum of 3 years in integrated care and/or healthcare environments
- Doctoral level education (preferred) in behavioral health, health care administration, or primary care
- Masters level education in behavioral health or health care administration
- Healthcare executive training programs/education (e.g.: degree or certificate)

CERTIFICATES, LICENSES, REGISTRATIONS
- Healthcare executive training programs/education (e.g.: degree or certificate)
- Integrated behavioral health or healthcare certificate training

If Supervision Responsibilities Assigned:
- Current state license and/or board certification in a behavioral health (preferred)
- Current state license and/or board certification in primary care specialty (Family Practice, Pediatrics, Internal Medicine, Psychiatry, Nursing)

CHAPTER 10
Training

> **BOTTOM LINE, UP FRONT**
> - Interprofessional collaborative practice and language training are lynchpins for delivering safe, high-quality, accessible, collaborative, patient-centered care. Provide this training to all medical home staff at a minimum. See Chapter 2 for further information.
> - Newly hired integrated behavioral healthcare (IBH) staff may require additional training, which may need to involve external subject matter experts. Consulting psychiatrists are the exception.
> - Outside of academic or other formal postgraduate training programs, there are only a few stand-alone training resources for the primary care behavioral health (PCBH) model. There are no known training resources for medical family therapy (MedFT) or co-located mental health outside university degree programs.
> - Regularly train all clinic staff on the role of each team member and the practice's standard workflow models for maximizing such services.
> - Training is as much about shaping employee and patient expectations as it is about re-educating them to use new tools for managing health.
> - Use formal training and consultation resources as well as self-directed ones, such as YouTube instructional videos and demonstrations.

Simply hiring a behavioral health professional (BHP) or reading the literature on IBH will not sufficiently prepare your organization to launch one of these programs successfully. Adequate staff training continues to be a barrier to successful integration. Training resources for BHPs and medical home staff in general are vital, but also limited in availability.[1,2]

TABLE 10.1. Types of Professionals Hired into Integrated Care Settings to Provide Behavioral Healthcare Services

Registered Nurse	Medical Technician
Professional Nurse	Psychiatric Nurse Practitioner
Clinical Health Psychologist	Clinical Social Worker
Clinical Psychologist	Consulting Psychologist
Mental Health Counselor	Psychiatrist
Professional Counselor	Marriage and Family Therapist

Table 10.1 lists the types of professionals who possibly could be used in IBH programs. However, we refer you back to Tables 4.1 and 9.1 for those models that have been the focus of clinical research and practice during the past two decades, and the associated training needs of those professionals. It would seem much safer to rely on types of professionals for whom training already exists, or who are easily trained in the formal models—again, to maximize your likelihood of program success.

> *Onsite training is likely to be the most helpful for your clinic and mental health staff. In our experience, the more BHPs train with "real patients" and receive "real-time" feedback, the better their skill acquisition and retention.*

STAFF TRAINING: BHPS AND ALL OTHER STAFF

Let's briefly discuss the training needs you may have to acquire for any BHP you hire. Most of the formal initial training for BHPs in IBH models rests within their specific graduate degree programs. Unless the prospective hires have prior training or supervised work experience in the integrated care model you launch, you will need to procure some level of onsite or offsite initial training, particularly if the end goal is to create a standardized service comprised of these providers that produce reliable clinical outcomes and return on investment (ROI).

Onsite training is likely to be the most helpful for your clinic and mental health staff. In our experience, the more BHPs train with "real patients" and receive "real-time" feedback, the better their skill acquisition and retention. Once they are outside of university degree programs, BHPs find that resources for them are scarce except for the PCBH model, for which there are a few online programs and in which other consultants and experts in this field offer training. Clearly, there are subject matter experts and consultants who may help train your staff onsite. In addition, the resources listed in the next section may be helpful for initial training if onsite training is not feasible or if your BHP has not previously been trained in a specific model of IBH.

Finally, consider providing your BHP with a book that provides practice recommendations and tools for the specific model of IBH you have chosen to launch (some are listed in the next section).

RESOURCES FOR ONGOING TRAINING

Webinars and Online Learning

- Center for Integrated Care: www.umassmed.edu
- Collaborative Family Healthcare Association: www.cfha.org
- Mountainview Consulting: www.pcpci.org/BHIP
- Morehouse School of Medicine: www.msm.edu/Research/research_centersandinstitutes/SHLI/aboutUs/behavioralhealth/aboutus.php
- Arizona State University's certificate program and CEs for training in integrated care—clinical and management: https://chs.asu.edu/dbh
- Arizona State University Doctor of Behavioral Health Program: https://chs.asu.edu/dbh

Self-Directed Learning and Informal Training Methods

- Online Program Manuals:
  - Patient-Centered Primary Care Institute Implementation Kit Library: www.pcpci.org/pcbh-implementation-kit-library
  - University of Washington AIMS Center IMPACT Tools: http://impact-uw.org/tools/
  - *Centers for Medicaid & Medicare Services Information Resource Center Brief*: www.medicaid.gov/State-Resource-Center/Medicaid-State-Technical-Assistance/Health-Homes-Technical-Assistance/Downloads/HH-IRC-Collaborative-5-13.pdf
  - *RESPECT-Mil Center of Excellence Primary Care Clinician's Manual*: www.pdhealth.mil/respect-mil/downloads/pcc_final.pdf
- Online Videos: For example, the YouTube channel NCR Behavioral Health (www.youtube.com/channel/UC0Ed1tM85MYvC4JKUOwcZAA) offers video demonstrations of full-length integrated behavioral health appointments with patient-actors who have difficulties changing their behaviors (PCBH model); and the Primary Care Shrink channel (www.youtube.com/user/nserrano4ME) offers podcasts and videos of brief teaching points and sample PCBH interventions.

- Primary Literature: Journals of interest include *Families, Systems & Health* and *Primary Care and Community Psychiatry*. Also read reports from other organizations such as RAND and AHRQ.
- Books: Consider
    - *Behavioral Consultation and Primary Care* by Robinson & Reiter, 2016 (Springer)[3]
    - *Integrated Behavioral Health in Primary Care: Step-By-Step Guidance for Assessment and Intervention* by Hunter, Goodie, Oordt, & Dobmeyer, 2009 (American Psychological Association)[4]
    - *Medical Family Therapy and Integrated Care*, by McDaniel, Doherty, & Hepworth, 2013 (American Psychological Association)[5]
    - *Integrated Behavioral Health in Primary Care*, edited by Talen and Valeras, 2012 (Springer)[6]
- Membership in Professional Organizations: Relevant organizations include The Collaborative Family Healthcare Association (www.cfha.org) and The Patient Centered Primary Care Collaborative (www.pcpcc.org).
- Continuing Education Activities: These might include attending professional conferences (see associations identified above) and can pertain to motivational interviewing and IBH generally, or as a specific model.

ADDITIONAL CONSIDERATIONS ABOUT TRAINING ALL STAFF

Mental health as a field elicits a whole range of images, from Tony Soprano sitting in therapy, to Dr. Phil or Dr. Oz directing callers and guests on talk shows, to Billy Crystal conducting therapy with Robert DeNiro in Hollywood movies. We see the mental health field portrayed variably across popular media, leaving us all, including patients, with a range of impressions. None of these are likely to resemble IBH. That is why training is needed for all team members, including administrative, clinical, and support staff.

Staff training must accomplish at least one fundamental goal: conveying that effective behavioral health in the medical home means managing *any* behaviors that affect patients' health. This training also must teach the medical home staff how to refer and discuss behavioral health matters in nonstigmatizing ways. For macro-level training ideas, see www.pcpcc.org/resource/progress-and-promise-profiles-interprofessional-health-training-deliver-patient-centered.

For training other clinic and nonclinical staff (i.e., those other than the IBH staff), there have been distinct movements to develop and promote training in team-based care. At the absolute minimum, train your medical home staff on collaborative care, "A general term for ongoing working relationships between clinicians . . . who combine perspectives and skills to understand and identify problems and treatments . . ."[7] (Figure 2.1). Although these training resources continue to develop, consider starting with a basic training for all of your medical home staff—one that also can be tied to job performance. Consider the Center for Integrated Care (www.umassmed.edu/cipc) for online training available on this topic. Also consult the Web sites we have included throughout this book, which comprise a wealth of resources on IBH and the medical home.

If you intend to create team-based care training resources internally, refer back to the core competencies for interprofessional practice in Table 2.2 and consult the original source at http://aacn.nche.edu. We recommend using pages 15–27 of that report to devise a brief professional training for all medical home staff. You can use the content to devise teaching points and use the lists of core competency skills as your evaluation criteria. Once your staff learns the four general skill domains, you can expand the program by applying these domains to each staff member's job performance.

ADDITIONAL CONSIDERATIONS ABOUT TRAINING PCPS

Once primary care providers (PCPs) learn about the impending integration and relevance of behavioral health to their practice, have an additional presentation/discussion (or an ongoing series of them) on the common psychological/behavioral health issues, family relationship issues, and health behavior change approaches (e.g., motivational interviewing) that are appropriate to attend to with the new IBH program launch. This could be done internally, for example, by your BHP, or externally through some of the resources mentioned earlier in this chapter. Teaching PCPs basic skills about how to attend to this aspect of their patients' health may lead them to be more likely to take interest in the new IBH service.

Finally, it is common for BHPs to develop and deliver a 10–15-minute initial brief for PCPs, nurses, medical assistants, and administrative staff addressing the specific model of behavioral health service they provide; how the BHP will benefit and work with the entire team; where the BHP is located; and how to refer to him or her. This type of briefing should be repeated weekly or monthly in whatever formal and informal methods match your organization's culture. Staff meetings and medical home huddles are low-hanging fruit for facilitating education and training and ultimately, culture change. See the next chapter for a process to acclimate your staff to integrated care.

References

1. IHI 90-Day R&D *Project Final Summary Report: Integrating Behavioral Health and Primary Care.* Cambridge, MA: Institute for Healthcare Improvement; March 2014. Available at www.ihi.org.

2. Blount FA, Miller BF. Addressing the workforce crisis in integrated primary care. *J Clin Psychol Med Settings*. 2009;16(1):113-9. DOI: 10.1007/s10880-008-9142-7.
3. Robinson PA, Reiter J. *Behavioral Consultation and Primary Care: A Guide to Integrating Services*. New York, NY: Springer Science + Business Media; 2016.
4. Hunter CL, Goodie JL, Oordt MS, Dobmeyer AC. *Integrated Behavioral Health in Primary Care: Step-by-Step Guidance for Assessment and Intervention*. Washington, DC: American Psychological Association; 2009.
5. McDaniel SH, Doherty WJ, Hepworth J. *Medical Family Therapy and Integrated Care*. Washington, DC: American Psychological Association; 2013.
6. Talen MR, Burke Valeras A, eds. *Integrated Behavioral Health in Primary Care*. New York, NY: Springer; 2012.
7. Peek CJ, National Integration Academy Council. *Lexicon for Mental Health and Primary Care Integration: Concepts and Definitions Developed by Expert Consensus*. AHRQ Publication No.13-IP001-EF. Rockville, MD: Agency for Healthcare Research and Quality, 2013. Available at http://integrationacademy.ahrq.gov/sites/default/files/Lexicon.pdf.

Appendix 10A. PCP Script for Introducing the BHP

The statement below may be used in order to invite the BHP into the exam room so that the PCP may use teamwork to finish the appointment with the patient and BHP.

"I'm going to call Dr. Shneebley in to help us. He specializes in these sorts of clinical cases, and I'd like him to put his head together with us so that we can do our best to help you with this."

The statement below may be used to initiate a warm-handoff to the BHP.

"I'd like to have Dr. Shneebley speak with you/evaluate you/see you today to see what he recommends. He specializes in these sorts of medical cases and I'd really like him to help us manage this together. He will probably spend about 20 minutes fully assessing the problem before working with you on some targeted solutions. Do you have time today to see him after our appointment?"

Variation 1:

"I'd like to have Dr. Shneebley speak with you/evaluate you/see you today to see what he recommends. He specializes in these sorts of medical cases and I'd really like him to help us manage this together. He will probably spend about 20 minutes fully assessing the problem. Then he and I will discuss how we should all proceed together. Would you mind if I have him come see you here while I move on to my next patient?"

(patient responds "okay")

"Once you two are done, he and I can speak briefly and we will all come back together to make a plan for you."

Note that these scripts are intentionally vague. The reason is to ensure that mental health stigma or any other social barriers to accepting behavioral health treatment do not prevent the patient from receiving the most appropriate care. Once the patient meets with the BHP, the BHP will usually disclose his or her credentials and role within the treatment team via a standard introduction.

CHAPTER 11
Facilitating the Transition Process to Integrated Behavioral Healthcare

BOTTOM LINE, UP FRONT

- Involve the primary care providers (PCPs) early and often in the process of developing your integrated behavioral healthcare (IBH) service.

- Having new behavioral health providers (BHPs) shadow your PCPs for a morning or afternoon clinic is the most effective way to help them learn about the PCP's practice and start developing a collaborative relationship with teammates.

- Local leaders' preferences and space capacities will drive the decisions about how to most efficiently incorporate the BHPs.

- A "population approach" derived from your business case analysis (BCA) is an excellent approach.

- Having the BHP and PCP work together using screening, case-finding, and schedule review is an excellent strategy to identify as many patients as possible who could benefit from IBH services.

- The art of "referral" by PCP to BHP is important for the success of IBH. This process should be monitored and used for feedback to PCPs to improve their referring skills.

- Available, bidirectional, written (in a shared record), and verbal BHP-PCP communication is critical for achieving the goals of ongoing integrated and collaborative care.

- Continuity of care over time is an important characteristic of the Patient-Centered Medical Home (PCMH) model and should be key for the primary care behavioral health (PCBH) model as well. Both PCPs and BHPs (when appropriate) can have longitudinal relationships with patients that vary in intensity according to their medical and mental health needs.

In Chapter 4, we described models of integrated care, summarizing the structure and function of each to help you understand the range of professionals you might hire and programs you might develop. In Chapters 5–7, we explained how to run the business side of these models. In this chapter we delve into how these work in action.

Getting everyone to work together in pursuit of shared goals can be challenging. This chapter describes a process intended to help you facilitate expectations, adaptation, and acclimation to integrated care among all of your staff. Because an effective process often is the difference between no progress and achieved progress, our focus is on clearly describing the transition process to integrated behavioral healthcare. Because PCPs' adjustment to and use of IBH services are paramount to success, most of this chapter is written from a PCP's perspective.

> *Effective process often is the difference between no progress and achieved progress. Our focus is on clearly describing the transition process to integrated behavioral healthcare.*

Begin the transition process by facilitating the right mindset among staff—PCPs and non-PCPs. Exchanging information through conversations and other activities helps educate and familiarize the entire staff with what may come. At the same time, you will learn more about their understanding of IBH. Give them opportunities to discuss and share their thoughts with the organization's leadership—this helps you uncover their learning needs. You might even have them participate in developing BCAs or other business planning to facilitate your staff's buy-in to launching IBH programs.

Then, conduct the self-inspection of your organization to ensure you have the site license, electronic health record (EHR), Practice Management System (PMS), databases, and other prerequisites to start this work (refer to Figure 6.1, Chapters 6 and 7, and Appendix 7F). Cover all of these things first and help staff understand how the steps listed in Figure 6.1 influence your range of options for IBH programs.

GETTING TO KNOW ONE ANOTHER

Next, begin developing staff relationships that are likely to enhance delivery of IBH services. Without these positive relationships, and in the absence of deliberate efforts to help your culture change, integration efforts may not be as successful as you would like. They might even fail. Facilitating integration works a bit like a middle school dance—orchestrating awkward interaction, knowing it will improve

Chapter 11—Facilitating the Transition Process to Integrated Behavioral Healthcare

as people adapt to the demands of the circumstance. But unlike the middle school dance, you can do many things to mitigate the awkwardness of the experience by providing information about these IBH models, specific role descriptions for your staff, workflow models, and explicit tasks, such as shadowing.

When introducing a new service in a medical home practice, the leadership needs to promote the effort in a positive and informative way. Respected practice leaders should have information and discussion meetings with the PCPs and the office staff. They might describe the scope of work BHPs can provide to the practice which, depending on the model you select, may include common mental health problems seen in primary care, including, but not limited to, anxiety, depression, bipolar disorder, and Attention Deficit Hyperactivity Disorder (ADHD); family systems issues (marital discord, parent-child relationships, caregiver roles); cultural and familial influences on how the patient manages a chronic general health condition; and substance use disorders. IBH programs are, and should always be, in a state of continuous improvement based on formal (data) and informal (anecdotal) feedback on how it is working for patients and providers. For more about program evaluation see Chapter 8.

> *Facilitating integration works a bit like a middle school dance—orchestrating awkward interaction, knowing it will improve as people adapt to the demands of the circumstance.*

Presenting details about how the system will work, outlining a few clear goals, and describing a few *key* expected behaviors that everyone will need to adopt will help make it more likely that teams will achieve "quick wins" early on. Arguably, the best method for teaching the PCP about IBH is having the BHP observe each PCP in multiple appointments with brief (under 2 minutes) discussions of each case after each patient leaves. This also helps the BHP learn about the PCP's practice style and patient panel. This also facilitates a positive, team-oriented relationship between the BHP and PCP. Of course, this means that PCPs must make themselves available for the shadowing opportunities.

Once hired, the BHP must become familiar with the practice. Ideally, some of the PCPs have met the BHP during the interview and hiring process, but likely not all will have. If left to chance, the BHP and PCP can pass like ships in the night for weeks or even months before they connect. To jump-start this working relationship and create the initial bond between PCP and BHP, have them work together for a few PCP appointments. The BHP shadows the PCP through a full visit with each patient. Between patient visits, they share information about their respective views about the patients, the patients' problems, and about how each professional would approach helping the patients. This interpersonal and professional exchange serves as a foundation for the future collaborative relationship.

The BHP should be able to ask patients questions during the visit and offer observations and suggestions to the PCP between patients. This gives the PCP an idea of what the BHP can contribute to the care of his or her patients. Likewise, the BHP sees how the PCP interacts and communicates with patients and how he or she detects and handles emotional content, mental health issues, and behavioral medicine issues. After observing and discussion only one patient visit, this bond can be forged along with the necessary understanding of how each clinician can assist the other and the patient toward better care.

PCPs are quick to recognize someone who can help them take care of patients. If this connection can be made in a face-to-face setting, the future of their collaboration is often assured and they will work to establish communication and collaboration plans that replicate the close collaboration they experienced while working side by side. To facilitate a reciprocal learning opportunity, there may be benefit for the PCP to observe the BHP conducting an IBH appointment. Of course, when conducting appointments together it is imperative to explain to the patient why two people are in the exam room. Appendix 10 includes several scripts PCPs can use to help patients understand the role of the BHP and help them feel more comfortable accepting IBH services. For patients who are new to integrated care, seeing multiple providers during the same appointment or within the same day may be awkward initially.

SPACE AND WORKFLOW: THEY'RE RELATED!

Space

An important area to address early in the planning phase is IBH clinical practice space. In the best-case scenario, the office design includes dedicated space for behavioral health evaluation, intervention, or even psychotherapy, depending on the model selected. Yet, this is seldom the case. Typically, you must identify or create an appropriate area for BHPs to see patients.

Any space can serve as a BHP room, including exam rooms and PCP offices, as well as rooms especially designed or set aside for BHP purposes. Using PCP offices can be a little touchy when the program is new and the PCPs are not accustomed to team-based care. However, when BHPs are brought in as described above, they usually are seen as trusted colleagues, which should negate any turf issues.

There are several ways to create space for delivering IBH. When BHPs are conducting clinical care, they may see patients in their own office/exam room or in the exam room in which the PCP is working. Alternatively, the BHP may go into the exam room before the PCP to check in with the patient, explain his or her role, conduct a screening for mental health or other problems, or offer assistance before, during, or after vital signs are taken. Or, the BHP may go in at the end of the PCP visit, especially if there is a warm handoff whereby the PCP is teeing up a referral to the BHP during his or her visit. PCPs sometimes ask their BHPs to join in the visit to provide perspective and input during the patient interaction—especially after a successful observation period as described above.

Because BHPs tend not to have exclusive nursing and administrative support, they need only one room, oriented as an exam room, ideally, so patients receiving IBH for a mental health problem don't feel that they are being treated "differently" than other patients. They do need space to conduct calls as well. Having the BHP's workspace resemble the rest of the medical home teams' workspace goes a long way in de-stigmatizing IBH. It is also crucial to locate the BHP as close to as many PCPs' exam rooms as possible, or simply near those PCPs to whom the BHP is assigned. Still, if there is no separate space available for the BHP, he or she can use a "swing" room, just as PCPs do.

> ***PCPs are quick to recognize someone who can help them take care of patients. If this connection can be made in a face-to-face setting, the future of their collaboration is often assured and they will work to establish communication and collaboration plans that replicate the close collaboration they experienced while working side by side.***

If you launch the co-located specialty mental health model, your BHP likely will operate using a classic 50-minute visit behind closed doors, with Do Not Disturb signs posted, a white noise machine, and the request to not be interrupted. If this is your IBH service, you will need to create space and resources that support this model.

However, we strongly recommend that when the BHP is in the office, Do Not Disturb signs and white noise machines should not be used. Rather, the entire staff should agree to contact the BHP only when consultation situations arise. Unlike specialty mental health, where the therapy room becomes an almost sacred space safe from interruptions, the BHP's office or exam room in integrated care looks, feels, and operates just like another PCP's exam room in the medical home. As such, interruptions, are expected, but should be kept to brief communications of need between PCP and BHP unless it's an emergency. This will be a challenge if you launch the co-located specialty mental health model.

The other models may not be so challenging to assimilate into the primary care clinic culture, which often includes some level of organized chaos, interruptions, and on-the-fly consultations. For example, if you are running the primary care behavioral health (PCBH) model, the space should be used like any other space in the clinic. An exam room or other shared clinical area will work well for your BHP. If you implement the Care Management Model, any space where patient care can be discussed via telephone (e.g., a shared office with nurses) is sufficient.

Irrespective of the model, sometimes the BHP will need more private space or space more conducive to seeing the patient plus a few family members. If this is not something you can accommodate regularly, work with your clinical staff to develop a contingency plan. If they want your BHP to address these types of patient issues, they will likely be motivated to help devise a solution.

Patients also need some education about IBH so they can align their expectations with your IBH and medical home. This alignment generally fosters higher patient satisfaction and more effective medical care. Teach patients how to use your IBH product line, such as same-day appointments, walk-ins, interruptions, and team treatment by multiple providers in the same room with the patient. Let them know that appointments in integrated care settings should be between 15 and 45 minutes, depending on the service delivery model. We encourage you to create printed materials describing your IBH services and distribute these generously across all clinic areas.

Workflow

Screening patients for common mental health issues can help identify those who would benefit from IBH services. This reimbursable activity can lead to earlier detection and problem intervention. It also could take the burden of managing several problems in one visit off the PCPs' shoulders if your BHP screens and flags these patients before the PCP sees them.

Screening

Do not set up screening procedures before you establish the service end to receive positive screens. Your system needs to determine the best clinical option at the lowest cost for additional screening or assessment for that patient. For instance, if a patient screens positive on pain by a medical assistant, a nurse might follow that initial positive screen with a more structured screening/assessment measure like the Dallas Pain Questionnaire. If the disease of choice is depression, once the nurse identifies a positive depression screen with a screener like the PHQ-

2, he or she may administer a PHQ-9. These are quick, free, and effective ways to decide how to direct workflow. They also can be used by all models of IBH.

Another way to initiate workflow for your BHP is to administer an instrument like the Patient Activation Measure (PAM)[1] to all patients, as it assesses patients' overall motivation to manage their health, giving the BHP or other administrator a sense of the patients' perceived motivation and health literacy. This type of population-level needs assessments will get your BHP working in a way that creates additional valuable work.

If your standard operating procedure after a positive screen is that your PCPs see the patient next, determine if the payer for your patient offers an initial evaluation template to be completed for which reimbursement is guaranteed. These tools can help your team determine who can screen/assess, what screening and assessment measures are recommended for use, and who needs to document the results in order to get paid for those services.

Strategies Other than Screening

If you decide that your BHP will screen, assess, or treat these patients next, you may have to bill for the BHP's work, just as you do the PCP's. As we discussed in Chapters 6 and 7 and several appendices (e.g., Appendix 7D), there are several codes that you might be able to use for reimbursement. Make sure the codes you use match the screening you implement and the integrated model you launch in order for this to work smoothly. Use Figure 6.1 to keep you on course with this business strategy.

Active consulting requires time to find cases, a guarantee that the BHP is available for curbside consults, and warm handoffs. For case-finding, BHPs can review the schedule of PCP patients coming in prior to their visit and use data in the electronic health records (EHRs) to identify those who are at higher risk for or have identified mental health or general health problems. Electronic medical records (EMRs) facilitate this by allowing BHPs to review problem lists, medication lists, previous notes, physical parameters like measures of chronic disease status, and social history related to family and work issues. This potential list of cases can be discussed with the PCP in the medical home morning "huddle."

This is a much more *proactive* approach than just sitting around waiting to be "called" by the PCP for an IBH need. It also allows the BHP to actively role-model for the nurses and PCPs, the situations in which IBH can assist them with patients' specific unmet needs. This also may help the clinical staff develop specific population health programs and improve health maintenance. It also will ensure you meet your productivity targets as specified in your business plan. The desired end-state is that PCPs recognize these opportunities and engage the BHP for assistance.

> "Oh, yeah it would be good for you to chat with Mr. So-and-So . . . he's had a real struggle accepting his Diabetes diagnosis and his adherence is poor too. Plus he's not getting along so well with his wife. Yeah—can you give him a call and tell him that I'd like for you all to schedule an appointment to see what life-style strategies we might target to optimize his diabetes management!"

Since many patients on the PCP's schedule have needs that might benefit from BHP involvement, BHPs can do this kind of daily schedule reviews or scrubs for two or more PCPs and move back and forth between them, actively looking for ways to help out. Statistics and experience prove that there will always be plenty of work to do.

Note that these are less-formal ways to increase use of your BHP. Formal ways tied to your business case analyses (BCAs) are also viable and important. But these informal ways help build the relationship, which the BCA and business plan may not adequately do. Moreover, consider that if you on-board more than one model simultaneously (e.g., PCBH and Care Management Model) you may develop methods of screening performed by the nurse, which then build the PCBH BHP's caseload, and vice-versa.

Workflow models may change over time as your IBH program matures, but the overarching goal is to create opportunities for the IBH service to become part of the fabric of how care is routinely delivered. You will know you've arrived when even the mere contemplation of ending such a service elicits a horrified expression on your PCPs' faces. As one apocryphal story about the Canadian effort to integrate psychiatrists in family doctor offices in Ontario goes: "The PCP was asked who he would rather lose from his practice: his consulting psychiatrist or his office manager? He immediately responded: his office manager, but noted that this would be a challenge, since his office manager was his wife!"[2]

WORKING COLLABORATIVELY: REFERRALS, COMMUNICATION, AND CARE PLANNING

One step in the development of an integrated care program involves PCPs and BHPs learning how they might work collaboratively throughout the entire process of care, beginning with the initial consult the PCP sends to the BHP and extending to ongoing management and continuous reciprocal communication. Facilitating this collaboration guarantees that your program will mature and evolve, meeting more complex patients' needs more easily.

Initial consultations generally are established in two ways: referrals and warm handoffs. A *referral* occurs when a PCP determines with a patient that BHP services might be useful. The referral is made through tools set up by the practice (see below for more on electronic methods) so a patient can schedule a future visit with the BHP. A *warm handoff* is made by a PCP to a BHP during or after the medical visit. Sometimes it even occurs before the visit, whereby the PCP wants the BHP's feedback about the patient beforehand so this information can be integrated into the PCP's assessment and treatment plan.

Three variables that may direct these workflow models are the acuity of the situation as agreed upon by the PCP and patient, the BHP's availability, and the time the PCP has to conduct the warm handoff. As such, leveraging the team in the medical home is important for facilitating warm handoffs.

On occasion, a patient will self-refer. Ultimately, ensuring you have a solid process for these patient handoffs is vital. Note that no-show and cancellation rates exceed 34% in some systems for IBH, particularly when same-day appointments are not available or when PCPs do not adequately describe the integrated care service to the patient, including the reason the PCP would like the BHP's input. By contrast, no-show and cancellation rates for IBH services are 9% and lower when IBH appointment templates are optimized and the "PCP pitch" for behavioral health services is on target (Corso, unpublished data).

Regarding the "PCP pitch" to the patient, PCPs should develop a standard explanation for bringing the BHP into the visit or referring (warm handoff or standard referral). An important byproduct of how well the PCP makes referrals for future visits is the "positive hit rate" of patients willing to actually follow up when the BHP calls to set an appointment. If the PCP and the patient have come to a mutual decision that the patient should see a BHP, and the PCP has described the process and whatever basic coverage rules will apply, then the hit rate will be high. The patient will be connected with the BHP and will attend the initial appointment.

We encourage you to help your BHPs see patients the same day as their PCP appointment or as soon as possible thereafter. The reason: patients may be willing to discuss a particular issue with a new person (the BHP) soon after talking with their PCP, but as time passes, they may quickly lose motivation. If the patient presents high acuity, same day or immediate referral to higher level of care may be required. But remember that in some states, same-day billing is an issue. Refer to Chapters 6 and 7 for more information.

Once the patient is being seen by the BHP, it is important for the BHP to communicate with the PCP about the patient's progress—usually after the BHP has seen the patient for each appointment. It's also important for the PCP to know the disposition of the attempts to schedule the patient—successful and unsuccessful. Knowing that the patient was no longer interested or misunderstood the reason for the referral or the services they would receive, that the patient sought and received care elsewhere, or that the patient improved and no longer felt the services were needed helps the PCP determine how to proceed at the next patient visit.

The following are important to effective collaboration and communication between the PCP and BHP on behalf of the patient:

- The BHP should share all medical notes with the PCP via EHR. Be aware of regulations surrounding doing this for mental health care.
- BHP notes must include at minimum: accurate diagnosis, planned treatment approach and duration, progress assessment, follow-up plans, discharge disposition at end of the IBH treatment. With regard to coding requirements, see Appendix 7F.
- If the PCP visit deals significantly with the mental health issue that lead to the referral, the PCP should forward or "cc" his or her notes to the BHP.
- PRN (as needed) access in addition to regular transmittal of progress notes by both providers is critical. Providers should have each other's e-mail, office phone, cell phone, and pager information.
- Frequent feedback from BHPs should improve the PCP's ability to accurately identify and manage mental health problems without the BHP. Anecdotally, at the University of California, San Diego, we received early feedback in our program from our BHP director that PCPs' referring diagnoses were "inaccurate" about 50% of the time! This brings up a management point, and that is whether BHPs have the ability, right, and/or expectation to correct or edit the problem list for the BH-related diagnoses. We recommend that they do.
- A joint or shared "care plan" should be developed for the patient's general or mental health condition. Not only does documentation occur in the same place when possible, but recommendations from both providers support one another.
- The BHP and PCP each reinforce the recommendations of the other provider when seeing the patient for follow-up care.
- The providers should feel a sense of mutual "ownership" of jointly managed patients. This is operationalized in the ongoing relationship with the patient by the BHP as well as the PCP. There is evidence that this relationship has significant impact on concrete medical outcomes.[3]
- Visits with the PCP and BHP can be alternated and tapered with either provider.

A FEW WORDS ABOUT NATIONAL COMMITTEE ON QUALITY ASSURANCE (NCQA) RECOGNITION AND BEHAVIORAL HEALTH

If your medical home achieved NCQA recognition for PCMH before the 2014 criteria were released, your current IBH program may not meet the current criteria and, consequently, you may have a negative outcome when you next

TABLE 11.1. Progression of Behavioral Health Elements in NCQA PCMH Requirements 2008–2014

PCMH Application Section	2008 Behavioral Health Content
2008 Behavioral Health Content	
PPC2: Patient Tracking and Registry Functions	The clinically important conditions are chronic or recurring conditions that the practice sees, such as otitis media, asthma, diabetes, or congestive heart failure.
PPC3: Care Management Element B: Preventive Service Clinician Reminders	There is brief mention of "depression" as follows: Age-appropriate risk assessments (e.g., smoking, diet, depression).
2011 Behavioral Health Content	
PCMH 1: Access and Continuity Element G: Practice Organization	Factor 5: Training and assigning care teams to support patients and families in self- management, self-efficacy and behavior change.
PCMH2: Identify and Manage Patient Populations Element C: Comprehensive Health Assessment	Factor 6: Assessment of risky and unhealthy behaviors. Factor 7: The practice assesses whether the patient or the patient's family has any mental health conditions or substance abuse issues (e.g., stress, alcohol, prescription drug abuse, illegal drug use, maternal depression). Factor 9: The USPSTF recommends: Adults: Screening adults for depression when staff-assisted depression care support systems are in place to assure accurate diagnosis, effective treatment and follow-up. Adolescents (12–18 years): Screening for major depressive disorder (MDD) when systems are in place to ensure accurate diagnosis, psychotherapy (cognitive-mental or interpersonal) and follow-up.
PCMH 3: Plan and Manage Care Element A: Implement Evidence-based Guidelines	The practice implements evidence-based guidelines through point-of-care reminders for patients with: Factor 3: The third condition, related to unhealthy behaviors or mental health or substance abuse, has been identified as a critical factor and must be met for practices to receive a 50% or 100% score, i.e. at least one identified condition must be related to unhealthy behaviors (e.g., obesity, smoking), substance abuse (e.g., illegal drug use, prescription drug addiction, alcoholism) or a mental health issue (e.g., depression, anxiety, bipolar disorder, ADHD, ADD, dementia, Alzheimer's).
PCMH 3: Plan and Manage Care Element B: Identify High-Risk Patients	Measurement plans need to include determining high-risk or complex patients and suggestions for such measurement include those with mental health comorbidities.

(Continued on next page)

PCMH Application Section	2008 Behavioral Health Content
PCMH 4: Provide Self-Care Support and Community Resources Element A: Support Self-care Process	Factor 6: The practice provides evidence-based counseling (e.g., coaching, motivational interviewing) to patients for adopting healthy behaviors associated with disease risk factors (e.g., tobacco use, nutrition, exercise and activity level, alcohol use).
PCMH 4: Provide Self-Care Support and Community Resources Element B: Provide Referrals to Community Resources	Factor 3: The practice provides treatment or identifies a treatment provider and helps patients get care for mental health and substance abuse problems, if needed.
PCMH 6: Measure and Improve Performance Element A: Measure Performance	Factor 1: Preventive measures encompass a practice's entire population and are not limited to specific measures for a practice's patient population with chronic conditions. The intent of preventive measures is that practices develop activities to improve quality of care for all patients in the practice. Examples of measures include: depression screening.
2014 Behavioral Health Content	
PCMH 2: Team-Based Care Element A: Continuity	Element A: A team is a primary clinician and associated clinical (including behavioral healthcare providers) and support staff who work with the clinician. Factor 1: The practice provides patients, families, and caregivers with information on the importance of having a personal clinician and care team responsible for coordinating care, and assists in selection process.
Element B: Medical Home Responsibilities	Element B: Factor 1: The practice coordinates care across settings, including for behavioral health. Factor 2: The practice provides information . . . including how to communicate with personal clinician and team (behavioral health) . . . Factor 4: The practice provides evidenced based care, patient/family education, and self- management support. Factor 5: The practice is concerned with the whole-person care, which includes mental healthcare. The practice informs patients/ families/caregivers how mental healthcare needs are met (i.e., by the practice or in coordination with another practice).
Element D: The Practice Team	Element D: MUST PASS All clinical members (including behavioral health) are members of the team and are critically important to patient-centeredness.

(Continued on next page)

PCMH Application Section	2008 Behavioral Health Content
PCMH 2 (continued)	Factor 1: Job roles and responsibilities summarize a team-based approach to care.
	Factor 2: The practice delineates responsibilities for sustaining team-based care, and specifies how care teams align to provide patient-centered care.
	Factor 3: Team meetings may be informal daily meetings or review daily schedules with follow up tasks. (CRITICAL FACTOR)
	Factor 6: Care team members are trained in evidence-based approaches to self-management support, such as patient coaching and motivational interviewing.
	Factor 7: Care team members are trained in population health management.
PCMH 3: Population Health Management Element C: Comprehensive Health Assessment	To understand the health risks and information needs of patients/families, the practice collects and regularly updates a comprehensive health assessment that includes: Factor 6: Behaviors affecting health. Factor 7: Mental health/substance use history of patient and family. Factor 9: Depression screening for adults and adolescents using a standardized tool.
PCMH 3: Population Health Management Element A: Patient Information Element B: Clinical Data	**Element A** Factor 14: the practice records the name and contact information for the patient's other health care clinicians providing care including behavioral health. **Element B** Factor 1: The patient's current and active problem list or diagnoses include behavioral health diagnoses. Factor 6: Assessment of risky and unhealthy behaviors goes beyond physical activity and smoking status. Factor 7: The practice assess whether the patient or the patient's family has mental or behavioral health conditions or substance abuse issues. Factor 8: Periodic developmental screening. Factor 9: Depression screening and referral as needed.
Element E: Implement Evidence-Based Decision Support	**Element E** The practice implements clinical decision support (e.g., point-of-care reminders) following evidence-based guidelines for: Factor 1: A mental health or substance use disorder. (CRITICAL FACTOR). Factor 2: A chronic medical concern. Factor 4: A condition related to unhealthy behaviors.

(Continued on next page)

PCMH Application Section	2008 Behavioral Health Content
PCMH 4: Care Management and Support Element A: Identify Patients for Care Management	**Element A** The practice establishes a systematic process and criteria for identifying patients who may benefit from care management. The process includes consideration of the following: Factor 1: Behavioral health conditions. Measurement criteria include: Factor 1: The practice has specific criteria for identifying patients with behavioral conditions for whole-person care planning and management. Criteria are developed from a profile of patient assessments, and may include the following, or a combination of the following: • A diagnosis of a behavioral issue (e.g., visits, medication, treatment or other measures related to mental health). • Psychiatric hospitalizations (e.g., two or more in the past year). • Substance use treatment. • A positive screening result from a standardized mental health screener (including substance use). Factor 2: High cost/high utilization. Factor 3: Poorly controlled or complex conditions. Factor 4: Social determinants of health. Factor 6: The practice monitors the percentage of the total patient population identified through its process and criteria. (CRITICAL FACTOR)
Element B: Care Planning and Self-Care Support (MUST PASS)	**Element B** Factor 1: The practice works with patients/families/caregivers to incorporate patient preferences and functional lifestyle goals in the care plan and updates plan. Factor 3: The practice works to provide community resources to assess and address potential barriers to achieving treatment and functional/lifestyle goals. Factor 4: The practice develops self-management plans; for chronic conditions; for barriers. Factor 5: Care plans are tailored to health literacy and language considerations when possible
Element E: Support Self-Care and Shared Decision Making	**Element E** Factor 2: Patients have access to educational programs and resources to support shared decision making and self-care Factor 3: Self-management tools are encouraged for patients to collect data at home Factor 4: Adopts shared decision making aids

(Continued on next page)

PCMH Application Section	2008 Behavioral Health Content
PCMH 4 (continued)	Factor 5: Practice provides health education classes with peer-led discussion groups or shared medical appointments; allowing access to multidisciplinary care team
	Factor 6: Resource lists are developed for the needs of the practice population; includes programs and services for self-care
PCMH 5: Care Coordination and Care Transitions Factor B: Referral Tracking and Follow-Up	**Element B** Factor 4: The practice integrates partially (i.e.: co-location with some systems in common) or fully (i.e., co-location with all systems shared) with behavioral health care.
PCMH 6: Performance Measurement and Quality Improvement Element A: Measure Clinical Quality Performance	The practice uses performance data to identify opportunities for improvement and acts to improve clinical quality, efficiency and patient experience.
	Factor 2: Examples of acceptable measures include: • Depression screening in adults or adolescents, or in patients with chronic conditions or comorbidities. • ADHD screening. • Assessment of behaviors affecting health, such as smoking status, BMI, alcohol use and substance use disorders.
	Element D Factors 1-6: the practice sets goals and acts to improve performance, based on clinical quality measures, resource measures, and patient experience measures.
	Element F Factors 1-2: practice provides individual and practice level performance results to clinicians and practice staff.

For more information see the following Web sites: NCQA: www.ncqa.org; NCQA PCMH: www.ncqa.org/Programs/Recognition/Practices/PatientCenteredMedicalHomePCMH.aspx

apply for NCQA recognition. In Table 11.1 we depict the progression of criteria requiring attention to mental health in the successive versions of the PCMH recognition process by the NCQA. The table includes only those criteria related to behavioral health. As we mentioned in Chapter 8, you may use the criteria to develop additional metrics for monitoring the IBH service. Monitoring such metrics according to these criteria make the re-application process easier and also keeps your IBH product line aligned with the goals of the medical home model and the Triple Aim of improved patient experience, better health outcomes, and lower healthcare costs.

Another example of the codification of attention to mental health issues is the formulation of the document, "Joint Principles: Integrating Behavioral Health Care into the Patient-Centered Medical Home."[4] The document details "a complementary set of joint principles that recognizes the centrality of behavioral health care as part of the PCMH" (p. 184) Consider reviewing this article.

Through such institutionalization of principles and accreditation standards, our primary care health system will be transformed to include behavioral health in its purview of responsibilities and in all services it renders. There also are financial incentives for achieving such recognition and practicing according to such standards. As this movement gains ground across the country, from academic centers, to Federally Qualified Health Centers (FQHCs), to military systems, to finally including all insured patient populations, truly integrated care will become the way we practice primary care everywhere.

References

1. Hibbard JH, Stockard J, Mahoney ER, Tusler M. Development of the Patient Activation Measure (PAM): conceptualizing and measuring activation in patients and consumers. *Health Serv Res*. 2004;39(4 Pt 1):1005-1026. DOI: 10.1111/j.1475-6773.2004.00269.x.
2. Personal communication between Gene "Rusty" Kallenberg and Nick Kates.
3. Saultz JW, Lochner J. Interpersonal continuity of care and care outcomes: a critical review. *Ann Fam Med*. 2005;3:159-166. DOI: 10.1370/afm.285.
4. Baird M, Blount A, Brungardt S, Dickenson P, Dietrich A, Epperly T, et al. The development of joint principles: integrating behavioral health care into the patient-centered medical home. *Ann Fam Med*. 2014;12(2):183-185. DOI10.1370/afm.1633.

SECTION III

Case Studies, Profiles, And Exemplars

CHAPTER 12
System Initiatives

BOTTOM LINE, UP FRONT
- There are many different ways to launch successful, sustainable IBH programs.
- A diverse array of organizations are launching IBH and they are not all necessarily launching the same type of program or taking the same process in program development and implementation.

This section lists program summaries of various systems which have recently implemented IBH. We selected these because of their various payment models, organizational type, size, and structure.

IMPACT[1]

This was a large-scale series of research trials across multiple clinics in five states. It had high control on what was delivered, and to whom. In many respects it reflects the best-case scenario with regard to the clinical results that might be gained using screening and the Care Management Model. The diabetes arm of this program also included a bi-lingual aspect of service delivery and was conducted with African American and Hispanic patients, which helped demonstrate program effectiveness in diverse populations. Cost offset and clinical improvements were successfully gained. Note that funding for this program may not be useful for you unless you intend to have research grants partially or fully fund your IBH initiative. Lastly, it lacks information about how one might sustain this program without research funding. Fortunately, Section II of this book *does* provide such information should you choose to develop a program similar to IMPACT.

Initiative Name	Improving Mood-Promoting Access to Collaborative Treatment (IMPACT) Research Trials
Brief Description	• 1,801 depressed older adults in primary care randomly assigned to IMPACT care or usual care. • 18 primary care clinics. • 8 healthcare organizations in 5 states. • 8 diverse healthcare systems • 450 primary care physicians

(Continued on next page)

Initiative Name	Improving Mood-Promoting Access to Collaborative Treatment (IMPACT) Research Trials
Outcomes	• Greater satisfaction with depression care. • Initial treatments are rarely sufficient—several changes in treatment are often necessary (stepped care). • Doubled effectiveness of care for depression (50% improvement at 12 months). • Effective for Black and Latino populations. • Improved physical functioning (SF-12 Physical Function Component Summary Score). • As depression improves, so does pain.
Healthcare Costs	• Lowers long-term (4-yr) healthcare costs—$3,363 less total cost over 4 years, including cost of IMPACT intervention. • Intervention patients had lower healthcare costs in every cost category (outpatient and inpatient mental health specialty costs, outpatient and inpatient medical and surgical costs, pharmacy costs, and other outpatient costs).
Key Model Components	• Screening and systematic outcomes tracking (e.g., PHQ-9) to know when change in treatment is needed. • Active care management to facilitate changes in medication, mental activation. • Consultation with mental health specialist if patients not improving.

Initiative Name	IMPACT Applications to Patients with Diabetes
Brief Description	• A series of analyses of the IMPACT model specifically in relation to depression in patients with diabetes tested applicability to Latino adults, a general population of adults, and older adults in the original IMPACT trials • Depression is twice as common among people with diabetes as in the general population and is believed to adversely affect the complex self-care activities necessary for diabetes control.
Outcomes	• The combined diabetes and depression care manager tested in the Project Dulce/IMPACT pilot was both feasible and highly effective in reducing depressive symptoms. Depression scores declined by an average of 7.5 points from 14.8 to 7.3 • The Pathways/Group Health Cooperative (GHC) study reported that mean depression scores were significantly lower at 6 and 12 months and that, over 24 months, patients accumulated a mean of 61 additional days free of depression. • The sub-analysis from the IMPACT trails of older adults with diabetes found that the intervention was a high-value investment, associated with high clinical benefits at no greater ambulatory cost than usual care.

Healthcare Costs	• Depression co-occurring with diabetes is associated with higher health services costs (50% to 100% higher). • The Pathways/Group Health Cooperative (GHC) study reported outpatient health services costs that averaged $314 less than the control group. The estimated cost savings was $300 per patient treated (e.g., an investment of $800 in depression treatment was offset by a decrease of $1,100 in costs of general medical care). • When an additional day free of depression is valued at $19, the net economic benefit of the Pathways/GHC intervention was $952 per patient treated. • The sub-analysis from the IMPACT trials of older adults with diabetes found that the intervention was a high-value investment. In the diabetes sub-group, in the first year there was a $665 increase in outpatient costs and in the second year there was a $639 cost savings. Total medical costs, over 2 years, were $869 less in the intervention group.
Key Model Components	• Project Dulce/IMPACT project added a bilingual, bicultural depression care manager to an existing diabetes management team. • Clients averaged 6.7 visits with the depression care manager. • Project Dulce included peer-led self-management training. • The Pathways/GHC study had specialized nurses delivering a 12 month stepped-care depression treatment program (initial visit followed by contacts twice a month during acute phase, decreasing depending on clinical response) beginning with either problem-solving treatment psychotherapy or a structured antidepressant pharmacotherapy program. Subsequent treatment was adjusted according to clinical response.

COLORADO ACCESS[1]

This initiative was a contractual arrangement focused on Medicaid patients and also had some grant funding in addition to Medicaid reimbursement. Uniquely, risk stratification was used to help codify the patient population and assign resources accordingly. The goal of this project was cost containment. Similar stratifications could be used in developing an IBH program based on variables such as clinical severity, illness burden index, and/or varying cost per patient per month or year.

Initiative Name	Colorado Access
Brief Description	• Nonprofit managed-care plan with contract as regional Medicaid HMO and Regional MH Carve-Out. • 64% of enrollees in Aged/Blind/Disabled Medicaid aid code. • Part of MacArthur Initiative and RWJ Depression in Primary Care Project. • Analysis of overlapping populations in two plans showed that 40% of people had a MH diagnosis yet only 33% had ever seen a MH provider, and for most, this was a one-time visit
Outcomes	• The focus of this analysis was healthcare cost; data not available on outcomes.

(Continued next page)

Initiative Name	Colorado Access
Healthcare Costs	• Emergency Department visits/1000: from 220.3 at 12 months pre to 163, 24 months post. • Office visits/1000: from 211.8 at 12 months pre to 358.2 at 24 months post. • Admits/1000 from 49.7 at 12 months pre to 37.4 at 24 months post. • Days/1000 from 232.5 at 12 months pre to 205.4 at 24 months post. • Savings of $170 PMPM, $2,040/year. • 12.9% reduction in costs in high-cost, high-risk patients.
Key Model Components	• Centralized care management in the plan, with telephonic, onsite in primary care or in-community care contacts based on risk stratification. • Care managers were nurses or MH specialists. • Registry to track PHQ-9, treatment adherence, self-management goals and progress, educational interventions, case management and comorbid disorders and treatments. • Focus on top 2% to 3% of population using Kronick risk assessment methods. • Three levels of risk stratification, based on PHQ-9, presence of psychiatric or medical comorbidities, high risk for non- adherence, psychosocial stressors and treatment-resistant depression.

AETNA[1]

Obviously the structure of this organization involves both third party payment as well as managed care which means containing costs for the insurer were a primary concern in addition to delivering quality care. This example highlights cost savings to healthcare systems which are comprised of more than just primary care services to include inpatient, outpatient, emergency, and mental health. This initiative also involved some level of grant funding.

Initiative Name	Aetna
Brief Description	• Integration with PCPs — Depression — Pediatrics — SBIRT — Integrated BH. • 64% of enrollees in Aged/Blind/Disabled Medicaid aid code. • Part of MacArthur Initiative and Robert Wood Johnson Depression in Primary Care Project. • Analysis of overlapping populations in two plans showed that 40% of people had a MH diagnosis yet only 33% had ever seen a MH provider, and for most, this was a one-time visit.

Outcomes	• 61% drop in PHQ-9 score between admission and discharge (45% have moderate to severe depression >14 on PHQ-9) • 48% of enrollees with major depression achieve PHQ-9 < 5 (remission).

Healthcare Costs	• Cost impact: reduction on completion (n=375)
	  — Emergency Department use 39%
	  — Inpatient care 30%
	  — Outpatient visits 47%
	  — Psychiatric visits 3%
	  — Psychotherapy visits 290% increase.
	• Net total cost savings 39%.

Key Model Components	• Health plan penetration
	  — Office identification by volume, diagnosis, and pharmacy claims
	  — Creation of virtual disease registry
	  — Initiative with employer groups and multiple health plans
	• Infrastructure-Practice models
	  — Quality infrastructure—EMR, registries, population management
	  — Facilitated implementation—PCP office implementation toolkit
	  — Web site: www.aetna.com/aetnadepressionmanagement/
	  — Role of office administrator- training module
	• Lack of utilization—adoption and persistency
	  — Academic detailing
	  — Office manager single point of contact
	  — Recurrent communication—E-mail reminders
	  — Community physician thought leader communications
	• Reluctant to refer to health plan care management
	  — Focus care management on facilitated access to BH
	• BH provider network issues
	  — Conceptual framework and training models
	  — Training BH and PCPs
	  — Incentives
	• Health plan integration
	  — Similar to provider integration and cultural issues
	  — Integration of BH and medical health data set and care management system
	  — Data sharing and privacy issues
	• Mental Health Financing
	  — Transactional reimbursement and claims payment systems
	  — Silos between BH and medical financing—carve in vs. carve out
	  — Lack of standardized reimbursement codes to support screening, case management
	  — Funding cost of integration

CHEROKEE HEALTH SYSTEMS

Cherokee Health System is a Federally Qualified Healthcare Center (FQHC) and Community Mental Health Center (CMHC) spanning 13 counties in Tennessee. It has a diverse payor system which provides it some diversity in risk and robustness of revenue streams. This system also provides a modest amount of patient appointments for uninsured individuals. Uniquely, Cherokee integrates a self-pay method for offering IBH to these specific patients (www.cherokeehealth.com).

Initiative Name	Integrated Care
Brief Description	• Federally Qualified Healthcare Center and Community Mental Health Center • 66,290 patients (24,653 Medicaid [TennCare] patients). • 45 clinical locations in 13 Tennessee counties • 604 employees (21 Primary care physicians, 40 nurse practitioners, 54 psychologists, 64 Master's level clinicians, 37 community health coordinators, 11 pharmacists, 10 psychiatrists, 9 psychiatric nurse practitioners, 2 dentists) • Payors: 14% private insurance; 15% Medicare; 40% Medicaid (TennCare); 31% of visits are uninsured patients

Outcomes	• After At Least 1 Integrated Behavioral Health (IBH) Visit:
	  — 28% decrease in medical use for Medicaid patients
	  — 20% decrease in medical use for commercially insured patients
	  — 27% decrease in outpatient psychiatry visits
	  — 34% decrease in outpatient psychotherapy visits

Healthcare Costs	• Compared to other regional healthcare providers without IBH
	  — Lower specialist utilization
	  — Lower ER utilization
	  — Lower hospital admissions
	  — Lower overall cost per enrollee

Key Model Components	• Behavioral health screening in every primary care visit • Integrated behavioral health in all primary care clinics (PCBH model) • Reverse Integration Model in its community mental health clinics • Psychiatry integration in primary care (Co-located model)

INTERMOUNTAIN HEALTH[2,3,4,5]

Intermountain Healthcare is a not-for-profit health system based in Salt Lake City, Utah, with 22 hospitals in Utah and Idaho, a broad range of clinics and services, about 1,400 employed primary care and secondary care physicians at more than 185 clinics in the Intermountain Medical Group, and health insurance plans from SelectHealth.

Initiative Name	Mental Health Integration
Brief Description	• 82 primary care clinics are mental health integration (MHI) clinics • Mental health teams include a primary care provider *and* at least one of the following: psychiatrist, psychologist, psychiatric nurse practitioner, social worker, or care manager • Regional managers collaborate to shift resources to meet the complexity of patient needs in various locations

Brief Description (continued)	• The senior management leadership provides direction and commitment to sustaining MHI; regional and clinic champions are identified to monitor quality improvements and outcomes • Culture has been changed throughout Intermountain so that team-based care is the standard, with integrated behavioral health as a core element • All team members can access and document in a shared medical record; there are also electronic methods of enhanced communication; centralized systems of data collection are used to monitor outcomes
Outcomes	• MHI clinic patients with depression were 54% less likely to use the emergency department compared to depressed patients in non-MHI primary care clinics • 53.1% of diabetic patients with depression in MHI clinics have good control over their diabetes compared to 47.5% in non-MHI primary care clinics • MHI clinic patients report improved overall functioning in life; 81% said they were hopeful they could get well or stay well
Healthcare Costs	• Depressed patients within MHI clinics had insurance claims decrease by $667 in the year following their diagnosis • Patients having one other diagnosis in addition to depression had only an 8% increase in average charges compared to similar patients in non-MHI primary care clinics who had a 90% increase in charges • MHI clinic patients have an overall lower rate of growth in charges for all services (except outpatient psychiatry and prescriptions for anti-depressants—indicating timely referral and treatment for mental health) leading to overall savings ranging from 30%-80%
Key Model Components	• All patients in mental health integration (MHI) primary care clinics receive behavioral health screening — Mild patients receive routine care with care management or peer advocacy — Moderate patients receive care management with additional mental health support or peer advocacy — Severe patients receive an assessment/consultation with mental health specialist and all other team members • Models used include PCBH and co-located specialty mental health services (psychiatry) • Services promote treatment adherence and self-management

EDMONTON SOUTHSIDE PRIMARY CARE NETWORK[6]

This exciting initiative was launched by a network of primary care clinics in Alberta, Canada, in just under 15 months. They transitioned most of their clinics from a co-located specialty mental health model to the primary care behavioral health model. The fascinating aspect of this case example is that Canada operates with a single payer system (government-funded healthcare), but it also has a private system that operates as well. This may be exactly what the American healthcare system may look like over the next decade or two. Therefore, how IBH works in this system may give us insight into how it may work in the United States in the near future. The goals of this project were to decrease wait times for mental healthcare and provide behavioral healthcare to a broader population of patients so that clinical outcomes (e.g., for depression) and quality of life for their patients could be improved.

Initiative Name	Integrated Care
Brief Description	• Government-funded primary care network of more than 14 clinics. • PCBH model was launched over a two-year period using an expert consultant trainer over two, 2-day trainings. • Patients had lower health status and higher anxiety levels compared to Alberta norms.
Outcomes	• 8 of 14 clinics showed decreased wait times for behavioral health services. • More than half of the patients included in the analysis showed clinically meaningful improvements on the EQ-5D-5L, a health survey that assesses five dimensions of health functioning. • 77% of patients showed statistically significant improvements in depression as indicated by improved PHQ-9 scores.
Key Model Components	• Includes 7 full-time BHPs and 7 part-time BHPs. • Most BHPs were mental health nurses (bachelor's level, with a few master's level nurses); a few BHPs were bachelor's and master's level social workers. • Several lessons were learned, including the importance of balancing program outcome evaluation with practical service delivery implementation; the importance of using solid, but feasible outcome measures for BHPs; and the importance of ensuring that PCPs refer more patients to their BHPs, particularly for general health conditions (versus predominantly mental health conditions).

THE PIEDMONT HEALTH GROUP

This exemplar is written in narrative form, as the initiative is still underway at the time of this book publication. Critical to our discussion is that this system represents the smaller healthcare organizations with a significant Medicaid population. Furthermore, the location of this organization is in a fairly rural area, where both competition and resources may be scarce. Piedmont proceeded with integrating behavioral health with the clinical benefits being their first priority. Only following its initial success are they now working to optimize it and build a sustainable, scalable program. While we don't encourage the separate behavioral health department structure of this model, nor the co-located specialty mental health model Piedmont implemented, we commend this organization for developing a program which has been anecdotally beneficial and worth their up-front investment. We suspect that it will evolve overtime as their medical home matures. Such is often the case in the current healthcare climate—that the maturity of the medical home bears some impact on the maturity of the IBH.

The Piedmont Health Group, LLC, located in the Greenwood, S.C., area, has five office locations and 18 physicians with three mid-level providers in the areas of family medicine, pediatrics, and neurology. The group offers imaging, lab, sleep center, occupational medicine, and counseling. The area population is approximately 70,000. As of this writing, they have not achieved medical home certification; however, application has been made with the expectation that this will be a real plus for all the services offered.

There really was nowhere to send mental health referrals, and if patients had a regular need for support, many had to travel 30 to 50 miles for weekly care. They would not continue treatment through the entire treatment plan, and thus there was a real need for local mental care. The physicians saw a need to address mental needs of many of their patients and decided to add counselors to the office. This was partially pushed by one of the Licensed Social Workers in the community who no longer wanted to deal with billing and other administrative issues. The department has now grown to five members or 3.5 full-time equivalents (FTEs).

The physician makes a referral to the department who then follows up with further screening and treatment on an individual or group basis. The counseling department functions well, reaching at least a break-even point and contributing to the overall practice overhead.

There was a real need in this semi-rural area; there is a little insurance coverage and a significant amount of Medicaid. The Medicaid need is great in the community since the amount of paperwork is significant and other practices choose not to offer services to those patients. One area of real benefit to the community and the practice is the affiliation with major employers, the City of Greenwood, and the school system. Employee Assistance Programs (EAPs) provide a number of patients. The school system not only refers students, but also teachers through their EAP. Some of the EAP programs pay a flat quarterly fee for access to and the services provided while others pay on a discounted fee-for-service basis. This program eliminates the need for significant paperwork with no pre-certifications necessary since this adds significant cost to the other payer programs.

While the EAP program had been a plus, many employers do not explain this program well and the patient sometimes is seen under normal insurance. There are limited resources in the practice for marketing and additional staffing so there are needs that remain unmet.

Beyond meeting the needs of the local community and employers, the real benefit has been the freeing up of time for the primary care provider. This has not been tracked but it has clearly been identified as a benefit to the practice.

The physician owners have agreed that this is a positive service to the community and have not worried about whether it is in itself financially viable. It is monitored regularly and it is expected that as the medical home model evolves, there will be an increase in activity in the counseling area.

References

1. Mauer BJ, Jarvis D. The business case for bidirectional integrated care: mental health and substance use services in primary care settings and primary care services in specialty mental health and substance use settings. Prepared by Healthcare Consulting; 2010. http://www.cibhs.org/sites/main/files/file-attachments/cimh_business_case_for_integration_6-30-2010_final.pdf. Accessed December 30, 2014.
2. About Intermountain. Intermountain Healthcare Web site. Downloaded November 17, 2015 from https://intermountainhealthcare.org/about/.
3. Healthcare Partners Medical Group. Enhancing Primary Care for Mental Health Patients—At a Lower Cost. www.accountablecarechoices.org/case_studies/enhancing-primary-care-for-mental-health-patients-at-a-lower-cost-1. Accessed December 9, 2014.
4. Reiss-Brennan B. How Intermountain Healthcare's mental health integration is improving healthcare. http://beckershospitalreview.com/hospital-management-administration. Accessed December 9, 2014.
5. Reiss-Brennan B, Briot P, Savitz L, Cannon W, Staheli R. Cost and quality impact of Intermountain's Mental Health Integration Program. *J Healthc Manage*. 2010:55(2): 97-113. http://search.proquest.com/openview/d396b1afe0278dc0f6f2695044a3ca1a/1?pq-origsite=gscholar. Accessed December 9, 2014.
6. Edmonton Southside Primary Care Network. Behavioural health consultant evaluation: Technical report. September 17, 2015. For more information about this report, please contact Jessica Schaub, Evaluation Manager at Jessica.schaub@edmontonsouthsidepcn.ca

Glossary

Accountable Care Organizations (ACOs)
Groups of doctors, hospitals, and other healthcare providers who come together voluntarily to give coordinated high-quality care to their Medicare patients. The goal of coordinated care is to ensure that patients, especially the chronically ill, get the right care at the right time, while avoiding unnecessary duplication of services and preventing medical errors. When an ACO succeeds both in delivering high-quality care and spending healthcare dollars more wisely, it will **share in the savings** it achieves for the Medicare program. (www.cms.gov/medicare/medicare-fee-for-service-payment/aco/)

Agency for Healthcare Research and Quality (AHRQ)
Produces "evidence to make healthcare safer, higher quality, more accessible, equitable, and affordable, and to work within the U.S. Department of Health and Human Services and with other partners to make sure that the evidence is understood and used." (www.ahrq.gov/cpi/about/index.html)

Behavioral Health Provider (BHP)
Licensed independent practitioners who are hired and integrated into the medical home in an integrated behavioral healthcare role. Typically excludes non-licensed independent practitioners who provide integrated behavioral healthcare (IBH).

Bidirectional/Reverse Integration
Typically limited in scope, breadth, and depth of integration. Its hallmark is hiring a primary care provider (PCP) to work inside a specialty mental health clinic. There is benefit to this model, particularly for patients with severe mental illness.

Business Case Analysis (BCA)
A decision support and planning tool that projects the likely financial results and other business consequences of an action. The analysis essentially considers "What happens if we take this or that action?" and answers in business terms—business costs, business benefits, and business risks.

Collaborative Care Model (also called a Care Management Model, Staff Advisor, or Care Facilitation)
Proactively targets specific diseases for which patients are being prescribed psychotropic medication in order to drive down disease prevalence, contain cost, increase treatment effectiveness and adherence, and access psychiatry consultation services.

Collaborative Family Healthcare Association (CFHA)

A nonprofit professional organization comprising a diverse membership of professionals including primary care providers (PCPs), researchers, educators, behavioral health providers (BHPs), and healthcare administrators committed to promoting comprehensive and cost-effective models of healthcare delivery that integrate mind and body, individual and family, patients, providers, and communities. (www.cfha.net)

Co-located Specialty Mental Health

A model in which behavioral health providers (BHPs) work at the same site as primary care providers (PCPs) which could be somewhere in the same building, floor, or even wing as the PCPs. This model lacks shared treatment planning, documentation, and provider goals; population focus; focus on general health conditions; and published quality metrics. It places the burden of collaboration on BHPs who may not have adequate training, skills, and buy-in to accomplish this.

Current Procedural Terminology (CPT)

A medical code set used to report medical, surgical, and diagnostic procedures and services to entities such as physicians, health insurance companies, and accreditation organizations.

Electronic Health Record (EHR)

Goes beyond basic charting and moves practices into improved communication and quality care while improving patients' abilities to self-manage and be active members of their healthcare. EHRs expand practices to reach beyond a provider's medical care to encompass other health professionals, interprofessional healthcare communication, and shared information systems with hospitals, specialists, and laboratories. They also are designed to be accessed by patients to improve their education and interaction in their own healthcare, meeting stages of meaningful use.

Electronic Medical Record (EMR)

Digital versions of paper charts that allow providers to document medical and treatment history, track data easily, and monitor baseline quality of care.

Federally Qualified Health Center (FQHC)

Includes all organizations that receive grants under Section 330 of the Public Health Service (PHS) Act. FQHCs qualify for enhanced reimbursement from Medicare and Medicaid, as well as other benefits. FQHCs must serve an underserved area or population, offer a sliding fee scale, provide comprehensive services, have an ongoing quality assurance program, and have a governing board of directors.

Health and Behavior Assessment and Intervention (HBAI) Codes
Current Procedural Terminology (CPT) codes for health and behavior assessment and intervention services that apply to behavioral, social, and psychophysiological procedures for the prevention, treatment, or management of physical health problems.

Health Information Technology for Economic and Clinical Health (HITECH) Act
Enacted as part of the American Recovery and Reinvestment Act of 2009 to promote the adoption and meaningful use of health information technology. Subtitle D of the HITECH Act addresses the privacy and security concerns associated with the electronic transmission of health information, in part, through several provisions that strengthen the civil and criminal enforcement of the HIPAA rules.

Health Maintenance Organization (HMO)
An organization that provides healthcare to people who make regular payments and who agree to use the doctors, hospitals, etc., that belong to the organization.

Healthcare Common Procedure Coding System (HCPCS) Codes
Often pronounced by its acronym as "hick picks," is a set of healthcare procedure codes based on the American Medical Association's Current Procedural Terminology (CPT).

Healthcare Effectiveness Data and Information Set (HEDIS)
A "set of process metrics used by more than 90% of America's health plans to measure performance on important dimensions of care and service. Altogether, HEDIS consists of 81 measures across 5 domains of care. Because so many plans collect HEDIS data, and because the measures are so specifically defined, HEDIS makes it possible to compare the performance of health plans on an 'apples-to-apples' basis." (www.ncqa.org/HEDISQualityMeasurement.aspx#sthash.Sk98CsqA.dpuf)

Institute for Healthcare Improvement (IHI)
A nonprofit organization focused on motivating and building the will for change, partnering with patients and healthcare professionals to test new models of care, and ensuring the broadest adoption of best practices and effective innovations.

Integrated Behavioral Healthcare (IBH)
Care that includes integrated treatments, program structures, systems of programs, and payments that focus on educating and motivating patients, helping them set goals, helping them adhere to any provider's treatment plan, and treating symptoms of any health or mental health condition by helping patients develop healthier behaviors, habits, routines, and thoughts. It also involves prevention,

outreach, educational, health promotions, and population health activities for all patients enrolled in the medical home.

Interprofessional Communication
Communication with patients, families, communities, and other health professionals in a responsive and responsible manner that supports a team approach to the maintenance of health and the treatment of disease.

Medical Family Therapy (MedFT)
Uniquely incorporates a stronger emphasis on patients' individual and social relational context in reference to their health and mental health. Like the Primary Care Behavioral Health (PCBH) model, it is also co-located, collaborative, and integrated within primary care. MedFT typically refers to marriage and family therapists who have received additional training in adapting their clinical skills to integrated behavioral health settings. They apply biopsychosocial systems theory to conducting psychotherapy with patients and their families who experience general health or mental health problems, including illness, trauma, or disability. These professionals may also provide more abbreviated care when time does not permit the specialty level of care. When time for specialty-based care is not available, these BHPs deliver a brief service more like the PCBH, with the addition of the social relational perspective mentioned above.

Medicare Administrative Contractors (MACs)
Multi-state, regional contractors responsible for administering both Medicare Part A and Medicare Part B claims. Centers for Medicare & Medicaid Services (CMS) relies on a network of MACs to process Medicare claims, and MACs serve as the primary operational contact between the Medicare Fee-For-Service program and approximately 1.5 million healthcare providers enrolled in the program. MACs enroll healthcare providers in the Medicare program and educate providers on Medicare billing requirements, in addition to answering provider and beneficiary inquiries.

Mental Health Parity and Addiction Equity Act (MHPAEA)
A federal law that generally prevents group health plans and health insurance issuers that provide mental health or substance use disorder (MH/SUD) benefits from imposing less favorable benefit limitations on those benefits than on medical/surgical benefits.

National Committee for Quality Assurance (NCQA)
A "private, 501(c)(3) not-for-profit organization dedicated to improving healthcare quality." (www.ncqa.org)

Patient-Centered Care
The patient experience is one of transparent, individualized, recognized, respected, dignified, and elected care related to one's own circumstances and relationships.

Patient Protection and Affordable Care Act (PPACA)
Commonly referred to as the Affordable Care Act, enacted to increase the quality and affordability of health insurance, lower the uninsured rate by expanding public and private insurance coverage, and reduce the costs of healthcare for individuals and the government.

Patient-Centered Medical Home (PCMH)
An approach to comprehensive primary care for children, youth, and adults. PCMH facilitates partnerships between patients and their personal physicians, and when appropriate, their family. Emphasis is on caring for populations, team-based care, and holistic care. Medical home is a similar variation of this model, but includes non-physician primary care providers such as nurse practitioners and physician assistants.

Patient-Centered Primary Care Collaborative (PCPCC)
A "not-for-profit membership organization dedicated to advancing an effective and efficient health system built on a strong foundation of primary care and the patient-centered medical home." (www.pcpcc.org)

Physician Quality Reporting System (PQRS)
A quality reporting program that encourages individual eligible professionals (EPs) and group practices to report information on the quality of care to Medicare. PQRS gives participating EPs and group practices the opportunity to assess the quality of care they provide to their patients, helping to ensure that patients get the right care at the right time. By reporting on PQRS quality measures, individual EPs and group practices can also quantify how often they are meeting a particular quality metric.

Practice Management System (PMS)
Assists with managing, scheduling, billing, and capturing patient data, while complying with the Health Information Technology for Economic and Clinical Health (HITECH) Act

Primary Care Behavioral Health Model (PCBH)
A biopsychosocial approach to population-based clinical healthcare that is simultaneously co-located, collaborative, and integrated within primary care. The goal of PCBH is to improve and promote overall health and mental health (may include substance abuse) within the primary care population. The hallmark of this model is that the BHP serves as a consultant to the PCPs and help patients

self-manage their symptoms. This does not provide a level of services equal to outpatient mental health (e.g., psychotherapy), and as such, is not a substitute for those services if they are needed. The BHP's schedule and practice style mirrors the PCPs' where each appointment is 15 to 30 minutes and up to 16 patients may be seen daily by a BHP. These BHPs also may provide curbside consults, educational classes for patients, or shared medical appointments.

Pro Formas
Describes a presentation of data, in financial terms, where the data reflect the world on an "as if" basis.

Relative Value Unit (RVU)
A measure of value used in the Medicare reimbursement formula for physician services. Medicare pays physicians for services based on submission of a claim using one or more specific Current Procedural Terminology (CPT) codes. Each CPT code has an RVU assigned to it which, when multiplied by the conversion factor (CF) and a geographical adjustment (GPCI), creates the compensation level for a particular service.

Return on Investment (ROI)
A performance measure used to evaluate the efficiency of an investment or to compare the efficiency of a number of different investments. ROI measures the amount of return on an investment relative to the investment's cost. To calculate ROI, the benefit (or return) of an investment is divided by the cost of the investment, and the result is expressed as a percentage or a ratio.

Specialty Mental Healthcare
Services that exclusively help people with mental illnesses (or are at risk for mental illness) conducted in outpatient mental health clinics/settings.

Substance Abuse and Mental Health Services Administration (SAMHSA)
The agency within the U.S. Department of Health and Human Services that leads public health efforts to advance the behavioral health of the nation. SAMHSA's mission is to reduce the impact of substance abuse and mental illness on America's communities. (www.shamhsa.gov)